Advance praise for College Mental Health 101

"Written with compassion and understanding, this book speaks directly to the 21st century college experience. Packed with a diverse array of personal stories and practical strategies, this book is a must have for anyone heading off to college."

—Yung Pueblo, *New York Times* bestselling author

"Easy to read, easy to navigate, and chock-full of quality information, *College Mental Health 101* is the go-to resource for any college-age student (and their parent) who wants to be empowered to navigate the journey toward mental health. I'll be recommending this book over and over!"

—Tina Payne Bryson, Co-author of *The Whole-Brain Child*,
Founder of The Center for Connection

"Mental health issues are on the rise for all age groups, and this is especially true for those attending college, most of whom are living away from home for the first time. Students must learn to navigate new challenges, some of which contribute to and exacerbate existing mental health issues. Parents are often uncertain about their role as their college-age child struggles with a new environment. In this remarkable book, Chris, Blaise, and Chelsie have provided an impressive amount of information to assist students, parents, college staff and counselors, and community mental health professionals to deal with the mental health issues seen on college campuses. They describe with great clarity different forms of therapy for a broad spectrum of mental health conditions, explaining the thoughts and behaviors that lead to a particular diagnosis. In addition to the wealth of information they share, what makes this book even more impressive and readable is the authors' writing style. Their clarity, empathy, and nonjudgmental approach are apparent on each page. Sharing their personal struggles and ways of coping when they were students, often with a sense of humor, conveys the hopeful message that mental health issues can be effectively addressed with the right support and treatment program. This book will serve as an invaluable resource to be read and re-read by college students and the adults in their lives as these students strive to be more hopeful and resilient."

—Robert Brooks, Faculty, Harvard Medical School (part-time),
Co-author of *The Power of Resilience: Achieving Balance, Confidence,
and Personal Strength in Your Life* and *Raising Resilient
Children: Fostering Strength, Hope, and Optimism in Your Child*

"This invaluable guide is for anyone navigating the complexities of mental health while pursuing higher education. Whether you're a student or parent, this book is like having a comforting, experienced friend with a roadmap to support you through each challenge with practical expert advice and compassionate insights. An essential resource to help students not just survive, but truly thrive, both academically and personally."

—Dr. Laura Markham, author of *Peaceful Parent, Happy Kids*

"The authors unparalleled insights into navigating the immense pressures of young adulthood—particularly the college transition—is nothing short of transformative. At a time when both students and parents face overwhelming emotional and psychological challenges, this guide is an essential resource. The authors' ability to address the often-overlooked psychological dynamics with parent, child in the high-school to college transition makes this work groundbreaking and truly invaluable for families seeking a path to success during this critical phase. Beyond the book, on a personal note, our foundation has worked very closely with Dr. Aguirre and we have witnessed first hand the practical ideas outlined in the book."

—Ryan Wolfington, Co-founder of Inspiring Children Foundation,
President of Jewel, Inc

"In this extremely well-timed and well-written book, *College Mental Health 101*, authors Christopher Willard, Blaise Aguirre and Chelsie Green address the mental health crisis on college campuses head on. They have created an incredible resource for college students, their parents, professors and coaches about the journey of emerging adulthood with mental health challenges. Offering a ton of great information based on research, years of combined professional experience and interviews with experts in the field, this book gives people the tools they need to navigate support services, classes, residential life, therapy, self-care and transitions to and from school. Alongside step-by-step guides, helpful exercises, sample questions followed by practical suggestions and clear explanations of diagnoses and treatments, the authors share many touching anecdotes from students and families as well as their own stories. I am amazed by how many practical, useful strategies and tools they have packed into this incredible book! I will certainly be recommending Mental Health 101 to my clients and my colleagues as a 'must-have' resource."

—Sharon Saline, Clinical psychologist, author and international speaker, Author of *What Your ADHD Child Wishes You Knew: Working Together to Empower Kids in School and Life* and *The ADHD Solution Card Deck*

"*College Mental Health 101* is my favorite kind of resource: refreshingly concrete and practical. This is exactly the kind of book that college students (and their parents) need. The authors answer hundreds of questions directly and honestly. How do I leave a voicemail for a therapist? What's the difference between college "partying" and a real problem with substances? What do I do when my roommate is really struggling? In a time when young people are sorting through so much information (much of it flat out wrong), this book will be a go-to—and a life saver—for many."

—Lynn Lyons, Psychotherapist and author of *Anxious Kids, Anxious Parents: 7 Ways to Stop the Worry Cycle and Raise Courageous & Independent Children*

College Mental Health 101

College Mental Health 101

A Guide for Students, Parents,
and Professionals

Christopher Willard
Blaise Aguirre
and
Chelsie Green

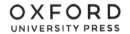

OXFORD
UNIVERSITY PRESS

OXFORD
UNIVERSITY PRESS

Oxford University Press is a department of the University of Oxford.
It furthers the University's objective of excellence in research, scholarship,
and education by publishing worldwide. Oxford is a registered trade mark of
Oxford University Press in the UK and in certain other countries.

Published in the United States of America by Oxford University Press
198 Madison Avenue, New York, NY 10016, United States of America.

Library of Congress Cataloging-in-Publication Data
Names: Willard, Christopher (Psychologist), author. |
Aguirre, Blaise, author. | Green, Chelsie, author.
Title: College mental health 101 / Christopher Willard, Blaise Aguirre, and Chelsie Green.
Description: New York, NY : Oxford University Press, [2025] |
Includes bibliographical references and index.
Identifiers: LCCN 2024044932 (print) | LCCN 2024044933 (ebook) |
ISBN 9780197764404 (paperback) | ISBN 9780197764428 (epub) | ISBN 9780197764435
Subjects: LCSH: School mental health services. | College students—Mental health. |
College students—Psychology.
Classification: LCC LB3430 .W45 2025 (print) | LCC LB3430 (ebook) |
DDC 371.7/13—dc23/eng/20250131
LC record available at https://lccn.loc.gov/2024044932
LC ebook record available at https://lccn.loc.gov/2024044933

DOI: 10.1093/oso/9780197764404.001.0001

Printed by Integrated Books International, United States of America

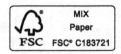

Contents

PART II. DIAGNOSIS

Introduction

Author's Note

In the winter of 1998, a phone rang at 3 a.m. in the Boston suburbs. It was me, Chris, one of your authors, as a 19-year-old college student, overwhelmed, exhausted, and crying, calling my parents. In retrospect, it was probably a panic attack made worse by lack of sleep and a few days of binging on just about every substance I could get my hands on.

My mom drove two hours down to my dorm to pick me up and take me home. By that time, I had settled down and clambered into the car to fall asleep and spend the rest of the weekend at home. I was lucky. My mom, a local psychologist who consulted many schools in the area, knew what to do. She gave me love and support, and she got me back into therapy. She also encouraged me to take a leave of absence. But, of course, I thought I knew better, and I spent the weekend sleeping off the panic and drugs, and then headed back to school to be with my friends.

Two months later, I was withdrawing from substances and on a medical leave, where I got a lot of the help I needed (thanks to a girlfriend who had cared enough to reach out to my parents—I still owe her my life). I was fortunate to have supportive friends, a knowledgeable family with no stigma, and the financial resources to support my challenges for the next two years before I went back to school.

And in some ways perhaps I was a canary in the coal mine. The mental health crisis has exploded across campuses in the 20 years since my leave of absence when I took time to "find myself and get my shit together."

These days, mental health crises are epidemic on college campuses, and I'm grateful to report that treatment and recovery are booming, too.

Luckily, I *did* find myself, I *did* get my shit together, and I *did* get better. Not only that, but I went on to become a psychologist myself, following in my mom's footsteps, primarily working with students and consulting countless schools around the world about their mental health programs. Yeah, things can get better. And when things are better enough, some of us want to give back.

That's what this book is about—written with two colleagues, including a senior psychiatrist who works in the world's best mental health hospital, Dr. Blaise Aguirre, and a younger social worker, Chelsie Green. The book is a compendium of all that we've learned as mental health professionals working with thousands of youth and families and, yes, as patients and students ourselves, too. This is a collection of what we picked up in graduate school and in books and at conferences along the way, as well as from our conversations with other professionals in the field. And most importantly, it includes what we learned while in conversation with students and their families.

Almost exactly 25 years after that phone call, our hope is that this can be the book that supports someone who might need to make that call, the recipient of that call, or better yet, that it prevents that call from ever needing to happen. We've seen many students recover completely and others who found ways to live fulfilling lives even with ongoing mental health challenges. We hope that this book supports more students to similar ends.

A Note to Parents

So you got that call home about your child's mental health crisis. *What do you do?* The most important thing is that you let them know that you care, and that you're there for them no matter what. As Chris's parents' therapist said when he was really struggling, "The number-one rule of parenting is never give up." This is likely the start of things getting better but also could be the start of a long journey. It's important to be prepared, and that's exactly what we hope this book can help you do.

Dr. Kelly Fraidin, MD, author of *Advanced Parenting* and the "Advice I Give My Friends" Instagram account, reminds us that all parents and caregivers have their default in a crisis. For some, it's to go into "mama bear mode" and protect, or maybe even overprotect. For others, it's to go into planning mode and call every resource possible. Still others get angry and blame their child, their school, friends, or even themselves. Others get sad, avoidant, check out, minimize, or deny. The more you know yourself, the more you can be there for your child so that your own "stuff" doesn't get in the way of their healing.

Getting your own support is key. You might want to find a therapist who will act as a consultant to guide you through this difficult time; they can help you be more effective, handle your feelings, or educate you about your child's struggles. Reach out to friends and family, especially if you know they've had their own relevant experiences and might have helpful advice or space to listen. You also might want to look up support groups for caregivers of those struggling with mental illness. Others in the family, like siblings, might want someone to talk to about what's going on as well, so be sure to check in with them, too.

Another challenge may be extended family or friends. Often when our child is diagnosed, we discover more about ourselves and our family of origin, and their mental health struggles, as well as what has worked or not worked well for them. This can be a rewarding process of self-discovery about your family's history, but you also might make disappointing discoveries, like that there is more blame or stigma than you expected. Other parents we spoke to reminded us you may also struggle with a partner or ex if they're not on the same page in terms of how to support your child. There may be awkward dynamics as well with stepparents trying to navigate their role. That's one of the many reasons we recommend that you as a caregiver have a point person—a couples or family therapist, or someone you consult with about your child's care that is knowledgeable, even handed, and supportive of different perspectives.

And so many experts we spoke with reminded us that, as a caregiver, it's not your job to do everything for your child but to help them build the network they need to succeed. Especially after the initial crisis, you might ask them more specifically what they want help with—is it finding a therapist, helping manage insurance, or something else? You can offer to help, but the best gift as a parent is to resist doing everything. Likewise, when they get to school and start reaching out for advice about friends and academics, we often feel palpable relief about our closeness and the level of trust they have in us. And yet, as Dr. Catherine Steiner-Adair reminds us, at this point in life, they should be reaching out to peers. We can listen and share *and* remind them to connect with their peers, too.

Indeed, as Julie Lythcott-Haims mentioned, collaborating to find resources at home or at school gives them the gift of agency and independence, and empowers them to be an adult who can take care of themselves—the adult we want them to be. It's a crucial part of their recovery to get them out of any learned helplessness—of having others always ride to their rescue. Rather than "swoop in and solve" (especially the minor stuff), "empathize and empower" them to engage the supports they'll need in this early part of adulthood.

And if you are the kind of parent who researches everything and anything—great, but remember, you're educating *yourself* on the issue, not educating yourself so you can lecture your *ahem*, grown child, on your newfound expertise. Nor is it appropriate to tell your child's therapist how to do their job. As our colleague Sam Himelstein puts it, you should be moving from manager of your child to consultant at this phase in life. And if you are setting out to educate yourself, read books and do real research. Don't just search Google or social media for advice.

The more you're able to listen (which is hard when you are so worried!), the more likely your child is to talk. The validation and support section in Chapter 7 has more on this, but the main thing your child needs is validation, not judgment; active listening, rather than lecturing; connection, rather than correction, so that they'll open up to you. They also need you to respect their boundaries and autonomy at this phase, and if you're ever uncertain, you can just ask them. Don't just call constantly but let them call sometimes; or you could make a plan and agree on how much they want you to be in touch and set reasonable limits around that. As your kids grow more independent, some of our own raison d'etre becomes less clear, and this is not the time to find it in rescuing your kids, or at least not in the same way. It's time to rediscover your own life, too.

You also might have to accept that you might not be who they want to turn to right now, and that's not only okay but developmentally normal and good. They're *supposed* to be seeking independence. A good therapist can help them get more objective perspective, but they may also gravitate toward connecting with an old family friend or relative who also had similar struggles. The more you give them space and permission, and encourage them to connect with anyone healthy, the better your relationship will be in the long term. We also realize that many parents are afraid a child will go to therapy and end up blaming you, the parent, or that you might feel jealous or even threatened by your child's relationship with the therapist. That's normal, too, and if you know you are feeling insecure, discuss it with your own support network.

You may want to set up all your child's care, especially if you're really concerned, and may wonder where to start. Many of the doctors we consulted recommended the family doctor or pediatrician as a place to start if you're at home, as they are often plugged into great referrals and resources locally. If your child is still at school, reach out to the health or counseling center. Tap into your other networks as well, perhaps other parents, but please do respect your child's privacy and ask before you reach out on their behalf. Some children have felt supported by their parents researching within their networks, while others felt like their privacy or autonomy had been violated.

And just as your child is eager to get back to school, you probably are eager for them to get back on track as well. Some of that might be fear of them "falling behind," or your own shame or stigma. Your child's recovery may be a slow, on-again off-again process, and your acceptance of that will be critical for all of you. Again, this is a great topic to discuss with *your* therapist or point person, because you don't want to push your child back before they're actually ready. Don't worry about the long-term future. You'll probably hear trite slogans such as "One day at a time" and "Progress not perfection," soon if you haven't already, and while they may be clichéd, they can be profoundly wise when embraced.

Even when your child is stabilizing, you may still be worried about them backsliding. This book is full of stories of two steps forward, one step back, and that's the reality. We don't recommend planning for things to go badly, but you may want to have an emergency plan in place. If your child does become a danger to themselves at some point, which hospital and doctor will you reach out to? Which and how many of the concerns described later in the book are signs that you might need to intervene? Do you have tuition insurance? Taking the time to consider next steps if things don't go so well will serve you so you aren't going into crisis mode yourself if that time comes.

And the last cliché is the airplane turbulence self-care one. Yes, you have to put your mask on first but also try to stay calm and breathe through this moment. Just like on the airplane, if the pilot is anxious on the PA system, the passengers will panic. But if the pilot can stay calm, then folks on the plane settle down. Calm is contagious. Of course, you *will* worry, but your child needs you to not worry so much they feel that they need to take care of you or to protect you from what is going on with them. Model self-care—go to your job, get exercise, drop what you need to for your child, but don't drop everything.

Welcome to the journey. The three of us have been on many sides of it. We know you'll all get through it and get through it stronger, with wisdom to share with your child, as well as your friends and family who may be going through this as well. Oh, and remember Chris's parents' therapist's advice, too: "Never give up!"

A Note to Educators

While this book is geared toward the students and families who shuffle in and out of your life every year, we hope that it provides some helpful resources for you to review, that it could be a resource that you share with the students who are in need of support, or maybe even something to assign in your classes.

If you're an academic in an institution, you might've been more focused on learning more about your field of interest, writing your dissertation, or conducting research when you were in graduate school. Learning how to support students who are having a mental health crisis was probably not a course that you took, and it's probably not what you want your main focus of your time to be. And yet you may just be in the perfect position to notice what's going on with your students because you, in a very real way, are the frontline worker for these students who have almost no adult contact at this phase in life. Other staff members only encounter a student experiencing difficulties when the situation reaches a breaking point, but you might notice if a student isn't submitting their assignments, excessively misses class, or otherwise seems "off." It might not have been the exact role that you signed up for, but it can be the reality of your position.

We know it might be difficult to know what to do if a student is struggling. Broaching the subject might induce anxiety of your own, so you might wish to avoid it altogether. Or you simply feel like you don't have the time to engage on this level, given the demands on your position. Or what if it's also just very much *not* your personality to listen, reflect, and empathize? (You'd be surprised to learn that some studies have found professors are just as helpful to talk to as mental health professionals.) Well, we are hopeful that this book can support you, too. Don't know what to do or say? You can always hand this book over to a student who is struggling, let them find some answers, and have them return it to you when they're ready. Rinse and repeat. And, in addition to this book, get a list of mental health resources available at your school or locally. Reach out to the health or counseling center to see if they have a list to share with you. This way, you will be able to easily point your student in the right direction (or even include some of that information in your syllabus to get ahead of things).

For other staff at institutions who might serve in roles that are more clearly related to supporting students and their mental health, know that as professionals, parents, and part-time academics, we want to thank you for your hard work educating and caring for our students and children, and for being frontline responders to this mental health crisis. You might already know plenty that supports your students, but this book might make a great addition to the wealth of knowledge that you already possess.

Remember that even if you spend plenty of time learning how to support students and do everything in your power to assist, it doesn't guarantee that everything will work out in the way that you want it to, or that it will wrap up easily. It doesn't always work that way for even the most seasoned of clinicians. But we hope that you take a moment to recognize your efforts and appreciate them regardless of what happens after your involvement—your contributions are worthy of praise.

How Did We Get Here?

There is an undeniable crisis in college mental health today. More students are anxious, depressed, binge drinking, and self-harming than ever before. More are flooding campus mental health clinics, overwhelming local providers, and entering college with an existing mental health diagnosis. In the past few years alone, articles in the *New York Times, Washington Post, Chronicle of Higher Education*, and others have described the college mental health crisis. When our colleagues Howard Gardner and Wendy Fischman at the Harvard Graduate School of Education recently interviewed thousands of students for a study on campus life, they found mental health came up more than almost any other issue.

In our professional roles, we've seen the reality of the college mental health crisis firsthand, but there are numbers that speak to it, too:

- Suicide is the second leading cause of death among young adults,[1] after overdoses.
- 60% of college students experience a significant mental health issue, with 44% experiencing symptoms of depression and 37% anxiety.[2]
- 67% of young adults do not seek treatment; this is higher for first-generation students and students of color.[3]
- 50% of mental health issues begin by age 14; 75% by age 24.[4]
- 64% of college withdrawals are due to mental health.[5]
- 26% of female- and 7% of male-identified students have experienced sexual assault,[6] with more experiencing sexual harassment of some kind.
- Students cite depression and anxiety as among the top impediments to academic performance.[7]
- One in three students seeks mental health counseling during college.[8]

It's our goal that this book offers hope and clear direction to the millions of college students struggling with mental illness, as well as to their friends, families, and professionals who are adjacent to this crisis. In this book, we give voice not just to other leading experts on mental health and education but to hundreds of students we interviewed about their experiences. Our hope is that we succeed in including a diverse range of voices from various backgrounds and college settings, and the people in their lives (both personal and professional supporters). And we've even included some of our own personal anecdotes and let our individual sets of experience inform what we've shared as well. This book is very much a product of a community coming together to support others on all things related to college mental health.

This Is a Big Book—Where Do I Begin?

There are many ways to use this book. You can read it cover to cover; in fact, maybe a professor has assigned you to do just that. But what we hope is that this book can just be a resource—you pick it up to read about a diagnosis if you're worried about yourself or another student, or you scan for tips on finding a therapist, learning about the hospital or medication, or whatever your questions are. We've organized the book into a series of a few hundred questions we hear the most. But it's not just our answers; we've added in voices of over 100 students, higher education officials, parents, mental health professionals, and more whom we've interviewed, to help you feel less alone. Not every voice will resonate for you or your experience, but hopefully some will resonate and help you feel less alone. And while this book is far bigger than we intended it to be when we started writing (sorry, Dana, our intrepid editor!), we know there is still probably a lot missing. If there's something you think we should have included, feel free to reach out to any of us, and we'll take notes for the next edition or a website we hope to build around this.

What Is Stigma?

If we'd written this book even a decade ago, we'd probably still be busting myths about depression, anxiety, trauma, and more, while spilling a lot of ink on issues like stigma. And yet, as we write this, a lot has changed. Maybe it was the pandemic, when we literally heard people say, "F—what anyone else thinks, I can't take it anymore, I need help!"

Maybe it was so many students seeing record rates of hospitalizations among their friends, or maybe the fact that so many young people as well as celebrities were talking openly on social media, but mental health issues are in the conversation like never before. And while stigma still has not been eliminated, and may still be an issue when you talk to your community, culture, or to older generations, things are changing rapidly for your generation.

The good thing about less stigma is that there is more good information than ever about mental health. The bad thing is that there's also more bad information about mental health and mental illness, and how to really manage it. We wrote this book to offer students scientific, research-based information about mental health from experts and scientists we've interviewed, combined with quotes from students and families who have *lived* through these issues to give you the best resources we can.

Where Else Can I Get Good Information?

Searching Google or asking an AI chatbot can help you find a lot of information, but much of that is misinformation or biased. Too many influencers and websites say that they have the "secret" to your never-ending happiness, but they are just trying to sell you an overpriced course, vitamin supplement, or medication you probably don't need. An online quiz might leave you thinking that you have a certain diagnosis that you actually don't. However, some resources available online can be supportive in your journey, whether they be more official or casual in nature. It's okay to do your own research, but do it well. The first things that pop up in your search are often the most popular, not the most accurate, and beware of influencers who may be motivated by money or sponsors. Remember, there are doctors and therapists out there who have a lot of answers, as well as research-based books. There are even scientific databases and journals to look at that your school probably gives you access to as well. Be thorough—this is your mental health we're talking about! We don't want to let just anyone or anything influence you.

But it's also easy to go down the rabbit hole and spend hours looking for the perfect diagnosis or treatment for yourself. If you're ending up with conflicting information and doubt, or it's worsening your anxiety, we encourage you to limit your time researching online if it's not actually helpful. And remember that our searches teach our algorithms in ways that we don't always want them to. Our online searches can lead to more advertisements and suggestions on social media for practitioners, groups, or influencers that may or may not be healthy, reinforce feelings of inadequacy, or make you feel like you will always struggle with your issues. Keep in mind, whether its suggested accounts or negative people, you can also always block or mute them.

Part of the reason that we wrote this book is to give you good information when there's so much out there and it can be difficult to navigate. It isn't possible to include everything and account for every nuance within our set number of pages, but we hope that it at least gives you a good place to start and continue your search for information from a balanced, accurate place. This book is a starting point, not an ending point, and a resource, not a treatment or diagnosis.

Why Me? Why Now?

One of the biggest questions students have about mental illness is simply "Why me?" Or maybe there are variations, such as "Why my brother?" "Why my roommate?" or "Why my child?" This is especially true when it seems like there was no big childhood trauma or adolescent drama, no warning signs that tipped us off, no indication that the high-achieving academic star who made it this far had any kind of struggle.

And yet, in many ways, the "why" doesn't matter. The three of us believe that it's often more useful to start taking care of your mental health than trying to understand exactly how it came to be, but it still can be helpful to understand.

What we believe is in what's called the "biopsychosocial model." Back when we were in college and high school, the debate seemed like it was always nature versus nurture. In fact, it seemed like we were constantly writing papers on whether issues were from nature or from nurture. Now we try to look at the *biopsychosocial model*; it's some combination of these that leads to mental health and thriving, or they contribute to mental illness. It's not just one thing, though; mental health and mental illness are multidetermined, multifaceted, intersectional, and more.

What Is This Biopsychosocial Thing?

First, let's consider the *biological* roots of mental illness. It might seem at first that there is not a lot we can do about this. It includes the genes you inherited that may have left you with a predisposition to mental illness. In fact, if you can, it's often helpful to make a family tree (or what therapists call a genogram) to look for patterns around personality, health, mental health, addiction, learning issues, and more, and see how close or far away they are in your family tree. If others in your family have struggled, reach out to them to see what has helped them thrive.

Other body factors matter, too, like how physically healthy you are. We're big believers in healthy eating, getting sleep and rest, minimizing stress, getting exercise, and those other factors. Of course, you should be taking medication if you need it, especially when you start the semester, and minimizing mind-altering substances. We know these behaviors are not exactly common or easy in college life, but, all kidding aside, are part of why so many students struggle with mental health in these years. So biologically, some of this you can change, and some you can't. This is about a third of why you do or don't have mental health issues.

And part of the biological is where you are in life. Like it or not, most mental health issues begin in the late teens and early twenties, so this is the highest-risk time statistically and genetically. This is when, if something is going to go wrong, statistically speaking, it is most likely to. But, in good news, if you treat and manage your mental illness now, it will be way less likely to be a lifetime, or even long-term, issue for you.

Not helping matters is that at the same moment in your life, it's one of the most stressful. Academic and social pressures, irregular sleeping and eating, and, yes, drugs and alcohol definitely increase risk factors. We know it's not what you want to hear, but more and more evidence is suggesting that the prevalence and strength of cannabis is contributing to the mental health crisis, not helping it. And while some things about your body and biology are tough to change, you can probably make some choices today for a healthier body tomorrow, in ways that will affect your mental health, too.

Then there's the *psychological.* Your brain and perception: Is your glass half full or half empty? What's your "cognitive style" in terms of how you perceive the world? Maybe growing up you had school or psychological testing, which says a lot about how you make sense of the world, and impacts your mental health and how you process the world.

And remember, like any illness or ailment, this is not about intelligence. Your GPA won't protect you from breaking your arm if you fall down playing soccer. SAT scores won't prevent cancer, or even a cold. Like any of those things, mental illness can just happen, to anyone. Wally Pansing, a dean at UPenn, reminds us also that it can come as a shock to students, friends, and families when a mental illness strikes. It looks even more out of the blue when the high-achieving happy "golden child" student in high school suddenly starts to struggle in college, and yet it sadly often has little to do with intelligence or hard work but is just a combination of factors that have been out of your control.

Many diagnoses also have cognitive effects, so you might not feel as focused or clear headed as you used to, but again with treatment those symptoms fade. At the same time, we can change our perspective and minds, and even rewire our brains, by getting the help we need. Consider some of the things you can do, some perspectives that have already begun to shift since learning more about mental health, and then consider how much more you'll learn in this book to understand and change your psychology.

Lastly, there are *social* factors. Consider your family, your childhood connections and caregivers, and the friends growing up who all influenced you. There are the losses, the moves, the bullying, the traumas, and the connections and caregivers. All of these shaped your perception of the world as well, and they are about a third of your mental health.

Adverse childhood events (ACEs) can impact you, and they might be worth reviewing (more on p. 215). And while ACEs can be depressing to look at, they are not a life sentence. In fact, there are also protective childhood experiences as well. Close friends, a sense of community, mentors, spirituality, arts, athletics, and, yes, your academics and smarts help, too.

Other social factors like race, class, immigration status, language, sexuality, and gender identity, and so many more also shape who you are, how the world perceives and treats you, and can make things easier and harder. And yet everyone is an intersection of various privileges and disadvantages; it's about learning to play the hand you've been dealt. So you can ask yourself, who has been a part of your social network, your support network in the past, as well as who is your community now, and what changes can make it one that supports your mental health?

These are some of the factors, some you may be stuck with, but when you pay attention to what you *can* change in these areas, you change how you feel and alter the trajectory of your struggles. When you face your challenges with radical acceptance of how things are, that's actually when you can start to take care of yourself and others, and get better.

When a student has a first "break" with mental illness, the question they and their friends and family often first wonder is, why me, why now? Parents or caregivers may wonder what they did wrong, when in fact we want you to remember the self-help slogan *You didn't cause it; you can't control it.* Students may wonder "Why me?" and yet another more helpful question may be *Why not you*? Mental health struggles are common, and very treatable, and if you've made it to college, you're clearly a young person who's capable of hard work and who has perspective and self-discipline that you'll need to recover from this challenge. You've made it this far, and we know that like millions of other students you'll make it through this challenge and graduate with a degree in experience managing mental health. And that's one of the most valuable things you've ever learned. It can help not just you, but countless others.

PART I
HELPING YOURSELF AND OTHERS

Chapter 1
Applying and Transitioning to School

Wherever you are in the college process, just beginning to think about it, or already there, thousands if not millions of students have been through the process of making a successful transition to college or back to college with mental health challenges. And hundreds of those students, families, and professionals have shared with us how they navigated that transition, and you'll find their voices here, answering some of the most common questions we hear. Whether it's picking a school, asking questions, or disclosing personal information in the admissions process, we've done some research for you. We've also made a timeline to consider how and when to get resources in place so you land comfortably, and we have explained how accommodations look different than in high school.

And while this is a time in life when you may want more independence, and to "do it on your own" without accommodations and supports, we believe this is the time to practice getting those supports set up on your own or with your caregiver. That's the best way to exercise your independence now, especially for the first year. After you've succeeded with those accommodations in place, you and your support team can explore which you might want to let go of at a later time.

How Do I Pick a School When I Have Mental Health Issues?

We feel lucky to have spoken to countless experts, students, and their families about how to go through the college search process while keeping one's mental health needs front and center. We also discussed other topics that might arise, such as taking a leave of absence, transferring colleges, studying abroad, and deciding when (or even if) it's time to return to school if you've taken a leave. We also want to acknowledge that not everyone has as many choices—your financial or family situation may end up limiting your choices, but still, here are some thoughts for the choices you do have.

As you start researching schools, the usual questions apply, but you have mental health considerations as well. Do you want a college that is big or small? Urban or rural? Close to or far from home? All of those are certainly important to grapple with, but let's think them over through a mental health lens. So let's consider the pros and cons of each, knowing there's not a right answer—there's only a right answer for *you*. We're just trying to help you think through pros and cons, and we are sure you'll come up with more than what we've laid out.

Should I Pick a Big or Small School?

Big schools may have more mental health resources than smaller schools. But it might be easier to slip through the cracks due to all of the bureaucracy or "red tape" to navigate to know who to connect with, how to access services, or even how to schedule a time to meet with your professor to find ways to stay on track or work on accommodations. Large state schools may go through more funding crunches than large private schools, which can impact resource availability. It may also be harder to find your support network at a larger school. Still, on the plus side, there might be more students struggling or who have faced struggles that you can connect with, and it's probably more common for students to be coming and going and taking time off, so there might be less stigma to face if you choose to do that yourself. Smaller schools, particularly private schools, may be easier to navigate but might have fewer resources. There are so many variables that we suggest to looking into the services and protocols at the colleges that you're considering.

Should I Pick an Urban, Suburban, or Rural School?

Urban schools may have livelier off-campus life, which means there is probably a broader range of supports off campus. This means more diverse therapists and modalities to choose from, local support groups for mental health issues, both formal and informal, that give you more choice and opportunity to "find your people." There are probably more informal community resources as well—spiritual resources, yoga and meditation classes, gyms, and up-to-date medical resources. Michelle Bowdler, author and former head of health services at Tufts, Brandeis, and Bentley Universities (which are all outside of Boston), reminds families that more diverse urban environments are more likely to have resources for LGBTQ+ students, and visibility may feel safer. Likewise, you may not feel comfortable being the only Black person around in suburban Ohio when you get groceries, or the only person in a hijab on a local bus in a rural area. In a city, you are more likely to see others who look like you, and this can offer comfort and relief. Similarly, medical resources like hospitals and clinics that can support mental health emergencies, or even work effectively with specialists who understand eating disorders or gender issues, may be more available in an urban setting.

The counseling center on campus is a good place to inquire about some of these questions, and you can always do so anonymously if that's more comfortable. Reach out to affinity groups on campus, or even identity-based alumni groups, for more clarity or advice regarding the specifics of the student experience or which resources are available. Sometimes it's best to get an unfiltered answer from students or alumni, especially considering college staff will most likely sugarcoat anything that might reflect poorly on the college. However, students and alumni can be particularly critical or speak from a singular experience that isn't reflective on the whole. So do your homework, gather as much information as you can from all sides, and see where that leads you.

Keep in mind that rural or suburban schools might offer a stronger campus community that is focused inward rather than outward. This may feel more supportive in that way with resources and community close by.

Should I Stay Close to Home or Go Far Away?

If you choose to go to a college that is close to home, it can mean your local providers (and prescribers) are close by, and there's a sense of familiarity.

There's less stress in finding your way around, and getting to know a local area's resources, whether that's grocery stores or hospitals. You can also head home easily if home is supportive, whether it's just to do laundry or get some rest, or to visit your home support network (like friends or teachers from high school, your old therapist, coach, or clergy). And you might want to just commute to school and live at home, which this option could provide.

However, a lot of students are deliberately trying to get away from home. Maybe that's from toxic dynamics in your family, traumas you've experienced in your old community, social and financial instability, or even caregiving demands and tricky boundaries. There's no "geographic cure" as such, but sometimes a fresh start really does make a difference. If you grew up in a big city, it might be comforting to live somewhere a bit smaller and slower-paced. If you grew up somewhere with a harsh winter that often makes you feel more depressed or down, a college located in a sunny and warm region is worth considering.

Should I Look Into a Public or Private University or College?

Public universities tend to be larger and include the benefits of a larger school. In addition, they are often significantly less expensive than private colleges and universities, which might pad your budget for therapy and other resources. However, some of what you are paying for with private universities are incredible resources, including accessible, well-trained clinical staff on campus or other student resources like accommodations and tutoring supports that can help if you're struggling academically. Given how expensive outside supports can be, you might actually save money utilizing campus services rather than paying a la carte for expensive private therapy.

Regardless, don't be fooled by the "sticker price" of a private university. If you come from a lower- or middle-class family, or have other siblings in college at the same time, your financial aid package might end up making a private education more affordable than a public one! (For example, one of the authors of this book got a $250,000 private education for $10,000 in cash and $15,000 in federal loans.)

What Kind of Housing Will I Want or Can I Get?

There's no getting around it: Campuses and residence halls tend to be loud and social environments, especially for the first few years. The reality is that even if you work on getting accommodations for housing, it isn't always guaranteed that the school will be able to meet your request to change your living situation, whether a single room or allowing you to live off campus. If you are able to fill out a preference form before you move in, advocate for yourself and ask for what you want. And be honest with yourself and the administrators about who you are—not who you want to be. If you think you'll suddenly transform into a teetotaler your freshman year (as one of us did), don't be surprised if you resort to your old ways and stay up late and party (which really annoyed that person's quiet roommates). If you end up in a less than ideal situation, you can always ask, but be forewarned, housing accommodations are rarely granted.

And while many students find the well-being, quiet, and/or substance-free dorms to be supportive and helpful, still others find them stifling in terms of building a social life or find they are more religious or less social than they'd like. It's a problem on college campuses that there are few living situations that are moderately social yet also reasonably quiet.

The search for an ideal housing situation may require some "radical acceptance" on your part, at least until you can choose your roommates/suitemates and your housing options, which often comes later in your time at college. Part of the transition into adulthood involves having to manage uncomfortable and often less than ideal environments and circumstances, and it may be that your first taste of this comes from the college experience.

Full Time? Part Time? Gap Year?

You might not want to go to college right now, or even at all. A gap year, as Dean Wally Pansing from Penn told us, can be a beautiful thing. You can have an adventure, earn some money, sort out your mental health, and give your prefrontal lobes another year to grow. You might worry you'll feel behind, but we've never met a student who regretted their gap year, and most come to college not just more mature, but full of interesting stories that make them much more interesting as potential friends when they do get to campus. There are many reasons a gap year is worth thinking about.

You also might want to do a partial gap year by taking a local class or two and working or volunteering. You could even enroll part time for your first semester or still live at home. In addition, there are a number of college preparation programs that might also be helpful over the summer, like College Semester Off, specialized preparation programs like at Landmark College, and others. As we say again and again, there's no rush! And as Dean Wally points out, "Education should be a pleasure, not something to survive. Take your time, enjoy it."

So How Do I Pick?

In the end, it all comes down to research, research, and more research. And while you may not want to reveal yourself by name to admissions when you inquire about services on campus, or share your struggles on an admissions essay or your interview, you can still find out the information you're seeking more anonymously. You can always call or email campus student services using a fake name, reach out to students or alumni from the colleges on your list, or ask your tour guide when you visit. Don't be shy! You are entitled to know everything you want to know; you are the customer. No question is too big or too small, and remember that you are considering spending years of your life at this institution, and potentially years afterward in debt to them. It's important that you feel that it is the right fit for you. Hopefully all of the considerations we wrote about here will help you navigate the research process, and worst case, you can always transfer if it ends up not being the best environment for you (more on that later).

Julie Lythcott-Haims, former dean at Stanford and *New York Times* best-selling author of *Your Turn*, was another wise and helpful voice we spoke with. Not only does she recommend choosing a place that has the best resources for supporting your mental health but also a college that has a culture of acceptance and understanding of mental health issues. Since you cannot fully rely on your home network, you'll need to make sure that your new community has the policies and procedures than can support you. She also suggests you find the support person on your campus who will be the equivalent of that teacher or staff you were closest to in school, your advocate. They might be in the financial aid office or in undergraduate advising, or they might be in athletics. It can be anybody, but you need to find someone with whom you can check in about life and they can help you navigate everything because they know the place better than you do. It may seem like college is just full of kids, but there are often hundreds, thousands of adults who work because they love young people; they all come to work to support undergraduates, not to get rich!

What Questions Should I Ask About Mental Health? And Where?

You might not want to bring these up on your tour or interview, but rather make a discreet call to health services or make an appointment to drop by if you'll be on campus for a visit.

Do they offer individual psychological and counseling services?

- Is there a limit to sessions per year or over four years?
- Can you keep the therapist you get?
- Is there a cost for these sessions? How much is it?
- What is the typical waiting time to be seen?
- How often can you be seen?
- What kind of diversity and cultural competence do treaters have?

Do they offer medication management?

- How often do you meet with your provider?
- Is there a cost associated with these sessions?
- What is the typical waiting time for the first session?

Do they offer group therapy?

- What sorts of groups do they offer?
- How do you sign up for a group?
- How often do the groups meet?

What kind of resources are in the community?

- Do you have therapists, hospitals, and prescribers you generally work with off campus?
- Do those community resources generally take student insurance?

Should I Mention Mental Health in My Admissions Interview or Essay?

We will be straight up with you on this one. We've gotten conflicting advice here. First, no college is allowed to discriminate based on your mental health history, but off the record, we heard different stories from folks who have worked in admissions. While it's absolutely illegal for colleges to discriminate based on preexisting mental health issues that may appear in your essay or interviews, we, and many consultants with whom we spoke, still urge caution in how much you disclose in the admissions process. That said, you'll never really know, and you might want to play it safe unless there is a real need to share. Also know, you're never *required* to disclose.

But *should* you disclose, even if you are not required to do so? Scott Marken, an admissions consultant based in Washington, DC, recommended that you not write your main essay on mental health struggles unless you try to own the narrative in an uplifting way. For instance, you might want to write about that rough semester during sophomore year when you started having panic attacks, but only if you also explain that you got treatment and there is a turnaround in grades that tracks with that. Still, you don't want to present that it's "over" either, as that might show that you're in denial of it being an ongoing issue.

Consider the purpose of the interview and application. You are trying to convince the college that you will be an asset to their community, so you will want them to have a positive image of you. In the same way that you would not highlight bad grades, fights with students, or skipping classes, you would not want to share the aspects of yourself that you do not feel are representative of who you are. If you are going to share a physical or mental health condition, do so in ways that enliven you, that highlight the obstacles that you have overcome in order to get where you are.

If you are considering including your mental health history on your application, how would you do so in a way that would make the college want you as a part of their community? What challenges have you had to overcome? How has it shaped you to be a more compassionate, active, motivated person? What does your diagnosis tell you (and them) about your grit and resilience?

You don't want a college admissions team to doubt your ability to succeed or perform well, especially under pressure or under the social demands of college life. Would they be concerned that you will not be able to complete any of your assignments and require lengthy absences? These days, many colleges are supportive of their students' mental health needs, and many provide on-campus resources and services. If you are going to disclose your mental health history, highlight the times that you have dealt with it, your sense of responsibility in knowing when to ask for help, and that you are aware of the resources that the college is providing.

Others we talked with suggested avoiding mental health talk altogether, or at least until you're admitted and want to pursue services. Some other consultants reminded us that you lose an opportunity to share something else important about yourself by overemphasizing your mental health journey, but it also is part of who you are, so you might feel moved to share that in your essay or in your interview. So with all of that in mind, we recommend that you proceed with caution until you've been accepted and then reach out to the appropriate offices on campus with whatever you need or want for support in relation to your mental health. Students themselves have a range of opinions and experiences. The important thing is to think it over carefully and consult with the people in your support network.

My experience with depression showed me that I can be in the depths of despair and that I have the ability to come out of it. It is part of who I am, and that I can make it. I would want a school that accepts me to know who they are getting.

—Aleesha, transferring from community college to a four-year college

I take medication that has helped me but that makes me feel very tired during the day. I always get my work done, but sometimes I fall asleep in class. It's not intentional and I am working with my psychiatrist to see if there are things that we can do, but I don't want my professors to think that I am being disrespectful, and I think that it would be important for them to know.

—Asa, returning to school after a one-year leave

Nearly everyone, or nearly every family, has someone with mental illness. I think that it stigmatizes people with a diagnosis when we don't talk about it. I bet you have many teachers and people in the admissions office who know someone with mental illness. Who cares if they know?

—Madison, high school junior

Planning a Support Network at School: A Timeline

Many students and therapists we spoke with recommend planning a schedule months out before heading to school to ensure what we call "continuity of care." Once you receive your college acceptance letters and decide which one you want to move forward with, it's important that you start planning what you need to do. Keep in mind that many college offices have limited hours or staff (or shut down completely) in the summer, so it can be hard to connect with someone if you reach out. Also know that during finals time (usually early May) the counseling and academic support centers are often swamped. For those reasons, starting the process of reaching out and making connections in April is key.

April

You've accepted a spot at your college (congratulations!). Now it's time to get started on the process of ensuring that you have the right support for your mental health when you get there. Talk with your home support team about your decision. If applicable, learn which medications can be prescribed across state lines, think about whether you need or would like to find an on-campus or local therapist, or if you will keep your therapist and maybe switch to seeing them through a telehealth platform. Likewise, decide if you'll keep your local prescriber and can get a semester of refills, or want to switch to a local pharmacy. (This might be required for some medications.)

Reach out to the counseling center and other student supports on campus to research local resources in your future college town. You might also ask where students go to do telehealth calls privately with their therapists if they have a roommate (some of our suggestions include empty classrooms, music studios, or library study carrels, though some colleges offer spaces for this specific purpose—ask!).

If there's a visit weekend for accepted students that you're able to attend, learn where the resources on campus are, and at least walk by to begin to get acquainted. Walk by the counseling center, gym, academic support center, dean's office, local pharmacy, and any other places you may utilize.

May

Reach out to therapists, prescribers, and others in your college town and "interview" a few of them if you are looking for new providers. See if they have the right approach, energy, identities, or other factors (including financial) that you're looking for by doing a short consultation (often providers will offer 15–20-minute consultations to answer any questions you may have and for you to see if they are a good fit). Set up your initial appointments for August or September when you plan to get to campus.

June

Be sure to find a local pharmacy if you need one or consider how to get your medications delivered. Reach out to the accommodations/disability support office and confirm what paperwork (e.g., diagnosis, neuropsychological testing reports, etc.) you will need for any accommodations you are requesting. In fact, get them the documentation even if you aren't sure if you'll use it; just have it on hand and ready to go if things get difficult later on. Your mental health provider(s) and/or caregivers should have the records and can help you send them over. Start role-playing self-advocacy with fake phone calls and meetings with your current caregivers to practice accessing services at college. Get any releases signed (authorizations for release of information or HIPAA forms) by your current providers now in case you need them to be in touch with your new providers or staff at your college.

If you have found out which dorm you'll be living in and have a chance to visit campus again, do it. Now that you know where you'll be living, it might be nice to see how long it takes to get to all of the resources you plan on taking advantage of, and to know your way around before you get there. If you can't get to campus, take the walk on Google street view to get a sense of it. Make sure you've reached out to the disability support office about any accommodations you are requesting, if you haven't already.

If you weren't able to earlier, book your first few appointments with the counseling center, therapists, academic supports, and any other providers and supports you need, if possible. We recommend afternoon appointments; you'll be surprised how quickly you adapt to the college schedule of being up late and sleeping late!

Start discussing with your caregivers and current team how much you'll want them involved in the transition, if you haven't already done so. Think about your red flags (Chapter 6) and when and how you'll want parents or friends to reach out to you if they are concerned about you.

August/September

When you get to campus for move-in day, walk around again and get a sense of where everything is in terms of the supports you'll be using nearby, as well as where you'll do your virtual therapy calls, if need be. Look over your weekly calendar and syllabi for the fall and consider when the stress points will be in the semester (usually midterms, finals, and any time a big project, assignment, or paper is due). If you plan to reach out to professors or your advisor about your needs, *now* is best the time, not during midterms or when things have gotten out of control. Go to the office hours and introduce yourself to professors and/or teaching assistants (TAs), even if you don't plan to meet with them regularly. Seriously, every professor we spoke to suggested to visit them during office hours, or even just say hi after class. They'll be much easier to deal with later if they know you now, and maybe you'll feel more comfortable reaching out to them if you are having a tough time. And there's no shame in scripting out what you want to say—they can definitely be intimidating people! You can try something like, "Hi, I'm Chris. I'm in your Psych 101 class and I'm excited about being a psychology major. I just want to introduce myself," or ask them for advice about how to stay on top of everything in the course. If nothing else, sit in the front row so they know and recognize you; almost every professor emphasized that they are so much more supportive of students who show up and sit up front than the ones they don't know who sit in the back and then bring up an issue in November.

This might also be a time when you think about how much you want to disclose to your roommates and new friends about your challenges with your mental health and any support you might want to ask for. But remember, friendships will change a lot that first semester, so be cautious about how much you share until you really have gotten to know folks (more on Chapter 3). Catherine Steiner Adair reminds us that this is also the time to really understand alcohol and drug policies, as well as understand consent and sexual assault policies and what you feel like are your values around these tough topics.

Keep in mind, too, that even the best laid plans don't always work out perfectly. The perfect roommate might transfer out, and then you end up stuck with someone who you don't connect well with. That perfect therapist that you found on the counseling center's website suddenly goes on parental leave until next spring. So much is out of our control, and all we can do is try our best to be present with what's happening in the moment.

What Can I Expect Once I'm There?

The other reality is that every accommodation that you request is not necessarily one that you will get. "Not everyone gets an off-campus single with a puppy and a gluten-free kitchen," as one social worker warned us. And yet that also means that college believes you can handle, maybe even thrive, with managing self-advocacy, the awkwardness of a human roommate, shared bathrooms, and some noise and disruption around you. You may find that you have more strength than you realized.

Our friend Lynn Lyons pointed out to us that there are enormous expectations going into college. Some of these are realistic, and some are less so. But one expectation many students have is that they will go to college and bring a different person or become a different person (like putting down a quiet morning person on our roommate form), but you will still be bringing your mental health needs. And so while college is a time of excitement and experimentation, you just may need to experiment more slowly than other students. Many students see college as an opportunity to try new things. And it is! But, when it comes to your mental health, your first semester or first semester back is absolutely not the time to stop or change your medication, stop therapy altogether, or stop other supports because you are having fun and have found some great friends. If things are going well, consider changing it up your second semester at school and after discussing it with the important people in your life.

Tina Bryson reminded us that students heading to college often idealize what the experience will be. While that's normal, it can create challenges when circumstances don't measure up. We idealize the place, the supports, and the potential friends, but we also can get disillusioned quickly when things aren't perfect. That's okay; we have a lot to learn from that process as well, and it takes time to find our balance and find that the supports we thought we could count on or need are different from the ones we are relying on even a few months in.

Unfortunately, you can't go to college expecting that everyone will support you. Hopefully, you will find some supporting friends, roommates, and adults on campus, but those informal supports are different from professional help.

It won't be and can't be the job of your roommate or new friends to wake you up, remind you about your medication and appointments, or confront you about your self-harm or substance issues. It's not even their job to get you to the dining hall or to class.

Lynn Lyons also reminded us that "College is about discovery and self-discovery—but don't forget discomfort is part of discovery." Discovering new friends means putting yourself out there even if you're a little shy or reserved and, yes, even if you have some social anxiety. Discovering your independence includes the awkwardness of sharing bathrooms and showers with others. Discovering your sexuality means new conversations about consent and pleasure with new partners. For most people these new things create discomfort, but discomfort and awkwardness do not always—in fact, very rarely—indicate an anxiety disorder or something else. Rather, they mean you are adjusting to the new people, places, and things and building new strengths, not falling into old anxieties.

Those first few months of sharing space with others *will be awkward*, and it's when many students start to wonder if they have anxiety, depression, or social anxiety. You might never like sharing space, even by the time you graduate. But if it's keeping you from showering or pooping or leaving your room or exploring friendships and intimacy altogether a few months in, then, yes, it might be an anxiety problem or is certainly worth chatting about with a therapist. And it's a hard line for therapists to draw—we don't want to minimize struggles and mental health, but we also don't want to jump to conclusions and "pathologize" a stressful few months. And so we do suggest that you might as well chat with a professional and get an outside opinion.

Likewise, the first months might or probably will feel lonely, and sometimes you will experience homesickness. These experiences, too, are more likely than not, especially when you've got a mental illness history, and they don't necessarily mean depression is about to return. Wanting to stay in bed could mean depression, and it could mean exhaustion, or mono, or avoidance, or a hangover, or a freezing New England morning, or feeling overwhelmed with all the new stuff you are doing. It could be anxiety, or it could be that you are meeting new people, facing new assignments, and dealing with new and scary things.

But the fact is, college is about how much there is to be learned, not just in your classrooms but in communicating about conflict with roommates, learning to share space with hall mates, and learning to meet new people in strange house parties with weird music and lights so loud and bright you can't hear yourself think, let alone have a conversation. All of this is hard. What you're learning especially, whether you have a mental health history or not, is how to be independent and to self-advocate.

How Do I Get the Accommodations I Need?

Our colleague Dr. Sharon Saline points out that when you're in high school, there's a structure and a path, and many adults have helped you build a routine—from classes and study halls, to homework time, to taking you to appointments, to reminding you of medications, even to providing you with well-rounded meals a few times a day. Things are laid out in more ways than we often might realize. But once in college, those structures fall away, and we are in charge of much more than we realize. This is where so many students start to struggle, especially those with neurodivergence or mental health issues. It's important to set up daily or weekly structures because of executive function challenges and because classes, activities, and sleep are less structured.

When you're struggling, though, many students often hate asking for help. Not only is it another thing to add to the to do list which is overwhelming, but it can make you feel like a failure, imposter, or super vulnerable because you have to reach out! But again, get those supports and keep them in place, at least that first semester. Go to the counseling center or academic support center and meet them, even if you've heard they aren't that helpful. Just check things out yourself. One problem Sharon sees again and again is students deciding to not get supporting services and setting themselves up to fail. Of course, it's easier to not try when you're down or the task feels too big. If you've written off the potential help, you are far more likely to fall into a negative spiral. As both Sharon and Julie Lythcott-Haims put it, you have to expect to show up for yourself. No one else is going to do it! Think about all the past successes you've had—many of which were in large part due to some of those accommodations that you now just need to practice asking for. Remember, if you needed support and structure to apply to college, you'll probably need support once you're there. There's no shame in that.

How Do Accommodations Work in College?

Public high schools are typically mandated under the Individuals with Disabilities Education Act (IDEA) to give supports, modifications, and accommodations to students. At college, it's about *equal access* and *banning discrimination* against students with disabilities, but there's no mandate for services. You have to register with the disabilities office, and remember they won't just know because you told your advisor or shared about it in your admissions essay. You have to reach out directly with the office.

Even once you do that, they are not mandated to make modifications to the curriculum, which is true in high school, where you may have been able to be retaught or taught ahead. Still, you can ask for things like extra time or note takers, but please know that *just because an accommodation is offered, it may not be helpful.* Extensions on assignments and incompletes often create more problems than they solve for many students, so know what really will help you and what might just bury you further. Likewise with flexible attendance policies, while it may feel easier to watch the lectures online, many students actually focus better in class and find they manage their time better when they do get to class, and with every good intention, never get caught up on the recorded lectures. Know yourself, don't fool yourself.

> When I was struggling with my final papers and a housemate told me to ask for an extension or incomplete, my mind was blown. Like it was this secret cheat code all the rich kids knew and so I didn't. So I asked, and my professors were super chill about it and gave me extensions. But I was still f—cking up—I'd get a new deadline and blow that, then I started taking incompletes, and so that by the time I should have been a senior, I had seven incompletes and no hope of graduating on time or meeting my major requirements. No one reached out to me or my parents or really told me, and I also didn't really ask. I actually had to spend an entire year including two summers catching up on ancient assignments and tracking down old professors to try to get work made up so I could graduate a year late. Don't be like me.
>
> **—Isaac, recent graduate with obsessive-compulsive disorder (OCD)**
> **and attention-deficit/hyperactivity disorder (ADHD) who**
> **successfully graduated with an English degree after five years**

We might have a different interpretation for Isaac than "fucking up," but if we'd known him then, we would have encouraged him to get psychological testing (see Chapter 5) and work with the writing center and other resources earlier. Still, for some students, taking extensions and incompletes is a blessing from heaven; for others, it's a disaster waiting to happen. Many experts suggested professors offer extensions in two-day increments and remind students of supports, and they suggested students ask for just short extensions themselves.

Remember, too, that getting class notes from someone else may or may not be helpful if their style is different from yours; a transcript is only as useful as you reading it, and preferential seating doesn't matter if you are struggling to get to class at all. Still, some accommodations you might consider asking for and that students we know have gotten include the following:

- Extended time or separate environments to take exams
- Extensions on assignments
- Note takers for class or assistive technologies (transcripts of class)
- Alternate formats for materials (e.g., video, audio for texts)

- Assistive technologies for writing (e.g., dictation software)
- Writing assistants and executive function assistants
- Preferential seating
- Flexible attendance and breaks during class
- Alternative assignments and assessments (e.g., oral exams rather than written ones to show your mastery of the material)

But you will only get these if you advocate and follow up with what the school asks you for. You may need documentation, and you may not get all of these, and it's rare you will get these after the fact if you've missed your window to get them in place. And remember that for some students, these accommodations may create more problems than they solve. This is another opportunity for radical acceptance.

Professors we spoke to reminded us that in college it's unlikely there will be extra credit for missed assignments, or that they will always be available on your schedule, and they aren't required to do these things. And a final is a final—the professor is not obligated to make a separate test full of new questions for you if you miss it or want to take it later, or to grade your late papers while they're on vacation. Too many students and families go in with the expectation that peers or adults have to be accommodating of their issues. But part of college is learning how to get the help and support you need. For better or worse, the onus is on you and your caregiver's family before you enroll to make sure you can handle what college requires of you academically and socially.

> Our family was really in for a rude awakening. Chad had an IEP [individual education plan] in place since middle school, but didn't want anything in place when he started college. After a very tough freshman year, we assumed he could receive the same services he had in high school for sophomore year in college. Even at a major public university, we learned the hard way he had to ask for dozens of things, only a few of which he got. We had to get [neuropsychological] testing all over again, too, at our own expense. Even though we were paying the bills, we couldn't ask his professors to let his advisor or us know that he was missing assignments, or even whether he was going to meetings with his therapist or writing coach. As parents, we were in the dark, and as a student, the supports we could get for Chad were a whole different ballgame.
>
> —Brian, father to a junior economics major with
> anxiety and executive function deficits

What Are My Rights and Responsibilities? What Are the School's?

Bryn Mawr has an excellent summary of the differences between high school and college regarding disabilities[1]

Process	K-12	College
What is the intent of the law?	Students are entitled to a free appropriate public education; qualified persons with a disability cannot be discriminated against.	To ensure that qualified persons with a disability will not be discriminated against and will have access—not entitlement—to academic programs and services
Who is covered?	Infants through high school graduates	All otherwise qualified individuals who meet entry criteria and who can document the existence of a disability as defined by the ADA and who have needs related to access
Central idea	Education is a right. Fundamental alterations of programs and services are required.	Education is an opportunity. Students must meet admissions criteria and be otherwise qualified. Students must also follow/meet other criteria of the institution such as health, character, technical standards, conduct code, and course objectives. No fundamental alterations of programs and curricula are required.
Identification	Schools responsible for identifying students	Students must self-identify.
Documentation	Schools responsible for testing students	Students must arrange for and pay for their own testing
Services	Schools responsible for any needed services. School must provide whatever services will help the student succeed in class. If necessary, schools must provide individualized tutoring.	Students must seek out services. Students are allowed only certain accommodations in college classrooms. Students must seek out tutoring, if needed, and must pay for it if the college does not provide tutoring for nondisabled students. Individualized instruction is not likely/guaranteed.

continued

continued

Process	K-12	College
Communication	Schools must communicate with parents at regular intervals about the student's progress	College is not permitted to contact parents without student's permission.
Accommodation arrangements	School must develop a formal plan, and it is the school's responsibility to track student growth.	Student must request and be eligible for accommodations *each* semester, and the student is responsible for much of the accommodation process.
Accommodation differences	Typical accommodations may include reduced assignments (requiring students to submit less work than others), extended time on assignments, grading changes (counting daily work equal with semester tests), test format changes, repeated chances to make a passing grade	No reduced assignments, extended time on assignments is usually at the discretion of the professor, no grading changes, no test format changes other than providing equal access, no extra attempts at tests; in other words, accommodations must be reasonable and must not compromise the rigor and/or academic integrity of the class

Going to college is going to be hard, and it is full of really difficult moments and decisions you must make and things you have to do. The more you prepare, as you're sick of adults telling you, the better off you'll be. And when it comes to getting the help you need, the more you know how to access it and advocate, the better off you'll be, too. Remember that parents and caregivers and past therapists and support will be less involved, and often not because they don't want to be, but they simply are not allowed to sign the forms and meet the deans and access the services that you'll need to do the legwork for. See it as another of those outside-the-classroom learning opportunities and the chance to practice more of the less fun aspects of independence.

Chapter 2
Should I Stay or Should I Go?

There's a lot to consider if your mental health issues started or reappeared while you were at college. Should you take time off and, if so, how should you best use that time? Should you transfer, or is that giving up? What about studying abroad? And how do you begin to best explain to people what has been going on with your mental health, without feeling like it's some kind of excuse? We'll dive into more of these questions in this next section, as well as hear from students about their experiences and how they came to the decisions they did.

What Should I Do If I'm Going *Back* to School?

The previous chapter focused on going to school, but we haven't talked much about going back to school if you've taken a leave, formally or informally. If you've taken a formal medical or mental health leave, then you may need to be medically cleared, get a letter from a therapist, or do a readiness assessment to rejoin the campus community. Different schools have different policies about what they require, and in our experience some may not even be legal. Still, if the school has recommendations or mandates, they are there for good reason, and we strongly recommend for your sake and safety you meet the recommended criteria to come back. You might also have decided to transfer; we'll discuss that, too.

When you do go back, things won't be the same. You won't be the same after what you've been through. Friends may have moved on, gone abroad, graduated, or changed up their housing plans, and you may discover that your lives don't mesh in the same way. Your self-care routine may be impacted by a different need for social time, a different relationship to sleep and substances, a different routine with more supports in place, and even a new course load or different major.

And yet our conditioning and the people, places, and things that "trigger" old behaviors may be hard to escape, and it's easy to fall back into old behaviors, roles, and routines when we return to a familiar environment. Chris returned to college after two full years away, hardly knowing anyone on campus, and yet found himself sliding back into old unhealthy habits within weeks. And while most students we spoke with were glad they took time off and glad they went back, none of them said the return was as easy as sliding right back in. Dr. Ilan Goldberg, a psychiatrist who founded and directs Semester Off, an innovative program in Wellesley, Massachusetts, for 17–25 year olds, recommends a "readiness assessment" before returning to college. "Getting clear about one's diagnosis, dialing in the appropriate treatment or treatments, and knowing which accommodations are available are *essential* steps to take before heading back [to college]. Also, serious thought should be given to the best living environment for the particular student as not every student, particularly those with extensive mental health struggles, is best served living in the dorms. There's no shame living off-campus or at home if that's what's best."

> I thought going back would be the same as the first two years, but it just wasn't. My friend group had moved on, I was still friends with individual people, but they weren't a group any more. The therapist I'd had on campus had taken a job somewhere else. I went to some local support groups in town for the first few months, but once midterms hit, I got too busy and they fell away. Once the cold and dark hit, my depression returned and I was back isolating in my off campus room that I'd wanted so badly, but now more alone than ever. It was so much harder than I thought it would be. I finished the semester, then ended up going home and transferring altogether.
>
> **—Darcy, senior majoring in psychology with self-harm issues who later transferred colleges**

Not every story ends with a transfer, however, or ends with backsliding.

Going back was hard. I was embarrassed, I didn't know who knew why I'd left, I hated having to come up with a story and wonder what random people thought. My friends knew, but it was those acquaintances I felt awkward about. Some friendships had changed and my new roommates were kind of random, but I reconnected with my improv group and mostly focused on school, and it was kind of a relief to have less social drama to deal with and mostly just be a student. I was coming off a great stable semester off where I'd taken a couple classes and had a cool internship at a podcasting startup, and having some perspective on the world bigger than college also helped me focus on what mattered. Taking time off was a hard decision, and coming back was hard, but it was worth it for my mental health. The most important thing though was working hard on therapy and myself while on leave, and then putting all my supports in place before I got back.

—Madison, theater major and graduate from a medium-sized private college with depression and attention-deficit/hyperactivity disorder (ADHD)

Just like starting school with mental illness, going back you'll want to be sure you'll have supports in place. Check in with everyone while you're on leave, especially friends and professional supports to stay in touch and know who's got your back now and when you return. You'll also want to think about self-disclosure with roommates, and whether going back to the same living situation is healthiest for you. Take a look at the list for "*How Do I Build a Support Network of People?*" in Chapter 6.

Change is hard, even change for the better. Keep in mind that just because some things have changed while you were gone, you have a lot of *new* opportunities for healthy, sometimes healthier relationships, routines, and living situations that you didn't even know about before.

What Happens When I Go on Leave?

If you take a medical or mental health leave (note: these are called different things in different places), there may be some recommendations or mandates of what you need to do before you come back. There seems to be a question of whether mandates for what you "have to do" are legal, but regardless, we strongly recommend that you follow what your school asks you to do before coming back. Typically these are things like actively engaging and progressing in mental health treatment, showing some other involvement in a school- or work-related activity, and basically getting better to the point that your mental health no longer interferes with your learning or others' learning when you do head back to campus.

And we also want to remind you that there is no rush. We know, it feels so urgent to get back as soon as possible, but having seen hundreds of kids make and not make it, the longer you wait, the more likely you are to make it through without more challenges. Pretty much every single student and expert we spoke with emphasized this point again and again.

> The worst decision I made was trying to get back right away from my leave. I went back for the spring semester after a two-month leave that started in October and was falling apart again by February. I left again almost suicidal because I felt like such a failure. From there I started a longer term IOP [intensive outpatient program], figured out medication, took ten months off, and then went back to school with new supports in place and finished no problem. Yes, I graduated a year and a half late, but it was worth it.
>
> **—Raphe, now a successful graphic designer diagnosed with bipolar disorder and substance use disorder**

What Are the Top-Three Things I Should Do on Leave?

Focus on your mental health; focus on your mental health; focus on your mental health.

Okay, Seriously Though, What Should I Do?

Most schools will recommend you stay busy and engage in therapy, and we do, too. We recommend staying busy at least 25 hours a week. That doesn't have to mean working; we believe therapy, exercise, and a class or two (academic or otherwise) in all of that time counts, too.

Staying busy also means trying to keep a semistructured routine, which many experts recommended. Even if you don't have a lot going on, try to get up around the same time, eat and exercise around the same time, and all of that. "Suit up and show up," which is to say, please don't stay in your pajamas on the couch or your childhood bedroom with the shades drawn, or we guarantee you will feel like a depressed teenager again. Please get out there as much as you can, to your appointments, to a job or volunteer gig if you have one, to a class if you're taking one, and to social events, even if there aren't many going on. Take a Look at What Is Real Self-Care? on Chapter 6, and remember you've now got the time; in fact, you are supposed to use this time for building healthy self-care habits and getting better. Make a calendar for the week, and try to see if you can fill at least 25 hours.

The first part of your leave should be focused on getting better and getting stabilized, and the time before you return should focus on getting resources back into place on campus, following roughly the timelines described in the planning for school timeline section on Chapter 1.

There are other decisions to make as well. Your childhood home might not feel like a great option, but you may or may not have resources to live elsewhere. Likewise, if your parents aren't together, deciding where to live is a stressful question, and we suggest living wherever feels most stable and supportive and close to your care. You also might want to go abroad or do another non-mental-health-related program while you're away—if you can afford this in terms of time and money and you're medically cleared, go for it. But if your therapists are concerned about you embarking on a big adventure away from your supports, we suggest you really heed their advice. We say more about going abroad on Chapter 2.

Be in touch with your family doctor or pediatrician. Drs. Mark Bertin and Dzung Vo, who work with teens and young adults, both reminded us that one of the best places to start or restart your search for resources back home is with your old pediatrician. They can make referrals to therapists, smooth the path of treatment, and may even be able to manage your medication until you find a specialist.

You might also ask friends from home for tips, or ask your home support network to help you find good resources nearby. If you are not sure about going back to your old therapist if you had one, that's fine—you can still ask them for other resources and referrals. Therapists won't be, or shouldn't be, offended by the question. They should understand you are in a different place in life with a different set of issues and want a different set of supports. We just want the best for you, including starting with a new therapist. Also, make sure you know your insurance situation before you go on leave; for example, can you stay on the school insurance?

My high school therapist was helpful with the stresses of high school, but when I took a leave from college, I really needed someone who understood my eating disorder. She actually felt strongly that I work with an expert and a nutritionist and my doctor, and had some great recommendations for my parents and me and wasn't at all offended when they reached out to ask him for help.

—Vanessa, back at college after dealing with bulimia and self-harm

And What Should I *Not* Do?

We don't recommend visiting school a lot, except for paperwork or official business that you have to take care of. It might be upsetting or distracting to go back often, which might take you off track. In fact, many schools won't allow you to visit campus or campus events like away sports games while you're on leave. We also believe you need to stay away from friends and other folks who aren't a helpful influence. Look, we aren't going to lecture you like your parents about your friendship choices, but you probably know who those people are. Stay in touch with people who are doing well and thriving and lift you up, not those who may unintentionally pull you down.

Should I Take Some Classes on Leave to Stay Caught Up?

One mistake we've seen a lot of students on leave make is thinking that a class or two at a local college will be easy. If academics have been going smoothly and you've got your treatment going, we say go for it. But if you are still really struggling with your mental health, or left school in part because of challenges related to executive functions, learning issues, or academic issues, you might think twice.

Without structure in place like other classes, the inspiration of classmates who you can study with, a nearby library where you can meet friends, and a regular routine, many young people struggle to be part-time students and find it difficult to make it to class and get their work done. It's an irony we've seen again and again. Having *less* to do and less structure seems like it will make school and other parts of life easier, but actually it makes it harder to get things done. Then the academic struggles lead to feeling worse, and mental health starts spiraling.

Assess where you are, and think whether a class really makes sense. Does it make sense to take pass/fail? Will the credits transfer? Would you maybe enjoy something else like just taking an art or cooking or meditation class for no grade at all? Doing something noncompetitive and without grades or judgments is great for your soul, and for your mental health.

On my leave I did a few different things. I finished the IOP [intensive outpatient program] I was doing in DBT [dialectical behavioral therapy], and then went down to just doing one group a week and one individual meeting a week. A psychiatric nurse helped me get the right dosage of meds. I worked at an ice cream store part time, did lots of yoga, and took an improv class. I suck at improv it turns out, but it was still good to keep busy and laugh. It was hard only seeing friends when they'd be home for break, and I kind of was casually seeing a guy I met at improv, but mostly just worked on myself and took it easy.

—**Alyssa, graduated in five years with a business degree**

What Kind of Leave Should I Take—An Academic Leave? A Mental Health Leave? A Medical Leave? Just Take a Semester Off?

This might feel confusing as well, because there are different kinds of leaves. An academic leave is something the school might make you do if you aren't maintaining a certain GPA or earning credits on schedule. But you should know that a lot of more privileged and savvy students avoid this fate or getting on academic probation by taking a medical leave or mental health leave, usually the same thing. That might be useful to do, because so often academic struggles are rooted in a deeper mental health issue. Some schools will then be more flexible about what goes on your transcript and will wipe away any lower grades if you choose a medical leave before the academic leave kicks in.

There also may be different requirements about coming back to school if it's an academic, medical, or disciplinary leave. While mental health doesn't typically cause discipline problems, most of the students who were caught cheating or plagiarizing who we've worked with did it out of desperation when they were already struggling. Still it landed them on probation or a semester leave. Likewise, substance use or possession can land you in disciplinary or even legal trouble, and everyone's judgment is worse under the influence as well. While most students who do drugs don't get in trouble, most of the students we know who've gotten in disciplinary trouble on campus were under the influence at the time.

You can also just take a semester off. If you are close to finals and your providers think you can make it through before you really need a break, that might be worth considering, but your mental health should come first, and again, school is for enjoying, not just grinding through. But because a medical leave may require that you are medically cleared, or that you take a certain amount of time before you come back, some students want that flexibility, though it might have other financial costs. The important thing is to make a decision in consultation with the professionals and people in your personal life who know you and your challenges the best.

If you have had ongoing struggles with mental health, it might make sense for your family to look into tuition insurance. It's not cheap, but it may help you recoup some of the financial loss from leaving school part-way through the semester, especially if you are going back to school after a leave.

While we have shared our experience and some voices of students we know, the decisions about staying and going and how to use your time are up to you. But—we can't emphasize this enough—please make them in concert with what your providers feel is best for you and your mental health. *Success comes from happiness and mental health, not the other way around.*

I Don't Think I Can Deal With Going Back . . . Should I Transfer?

Other students may decide, after some challenges, that transferring is the best option for them. Transferring is not an easy decision, but neither is staying, and they should each be an active decision. Each has major drawbacks, and if that feels unfair, you're right—it's absolutely unfair. But they also both have major advantages. What's important is that you really weigh the pros and cons of each, and figure out where you'll get the support you need before you head back.

The fact of it is, "There's no such thing as a geographical cure," as they say, and "Wherever you go there you are." Those sayings might seem trite or cliché, but they are true in that whatever you decide, your mental health issues will follow you; the key is to figure out where you can most easily thrive and access the support you need. You'll want to consider the same questions we reviewed in the section on choosing a college (see Chapter 1) in terms of supports available but also consider some other questions, too.

Will a new environment feel like a fresh start? Have local resources at your school been helpful to you in the past? You may know the resources on your campus and whether they are helpful to you.

Will friends be supportive of the changes you need to make, or might some old friendships hold you back in old patterns? Are there people, places, and things and other triggers at your school that make things worse or better for you? Did you experience a physical, sexual, or relational trauma and just want to start again?

How much stress will the transfer process be, in terms of applications, but also will the stress of a new environment and making new friends outweigh the benefits of a "fresh start"? Even simpler logistical questions like costs and transferring credits, and differing major and graduation requirements are important to consider. There may be advantages to switching to a local state school, but you also may now have to go back and take calculus and or other challenging required classes that will impact your stress level and mental health. What are the transfer deadlines, and how will transferring affect your hoped-for graduation timeline?

Aiden came out of a public high school with lots of support into a big state school because it had the specific major he loved. We didn't know what was happening for the first year and a half, but finally it was clear that he was struggling with his depression and academics, failing most of the giant intro courses for his major and staying in his room. He got into the cycle of isolation and avoidance he'd had in middle school, a doom loop with his depression.

He took a leave and moved back home, but was just as depressed as before. He struggled to keep a job, and make it to local community college classes. In retrospect, he could have used better structure at home. Aiden's therapist continued to recommend a small local liberal arts college where he'd had some clients. We got the application done and it was a total game changer.

He lived at home the first semester as he settled in academically and then got an apartment near campus. The professors and advisors were incredibly supportive and wanted him to succeed—they even let him take his exams orally because of his dyslexia. His prescriber and high school therapist were close by. It took eight and a half years from high school to college graduation but he did it, and we're incredibly proud.

—Ronald, parent of Aiden who is now working toward a master's degree in marketing

I have an older dad, and he was diagnosed with pancreatic cancer when I was a freshman, right around when I was struggling with own depression. I took the spring semester off to come home and be close by, then ended up transferring to a local college where I was taking classes during that other semester. My social time at college was going to be screwed up by the family issues one way or another with traveling home all the time, but being able to be twenty minutes instead of six hours from home really mattered to me. I don't regret transferring, even if the school didn't have the prestige of the one I'd started at.

—Anton, recent college graduate who now works in finance

Should I Do a Year or Semester Abroad or Away?

If your mental health has been stable and issues are being treated, there's no reason to prevent you from doing much of anything, including going abroad. Like going off or going back to school, you'll want to be sure that you have supports and resources in place before you go. A foreign country can feel extremely isolating—new people; new languages; different foods, cultures, and routines to get used to; different weather and schedules—all of these can overwhelm us and impact our sense of connection and stability. As long as you plan for these contingencies and care for your mental health, you should be okay. Look over your support list from earlier and see what you can put together abroad.

If you do have a therapist, you will want to get their opinion, and you may want to see if they feel comfortable meeting with you online, and if the hours work, assuming there is a time change. Not every therapist will work online; in fact, they really aren't supposed to provide services, even across state lines, so if yours doesn't, consider finding an online therapist who you do feel comfortable with. And not every therapist is as good online as in person. Try some sessions over video before you head out to make sure it works for the two of you.

You also might find a therapist abroad, but therapy as we know it really is a uniquely North American phenomenon. Still, different regions of the world do have therapists. They are often fewer and further between, but it could still be a very cool cultural experience to do therapy in a different language or culture. Bear in mind that different places have different trends. For instance, southern South America has a long tradition of therapy, but it is often very psychoanalytic and now increasingly mindfulness oriented. (Buenos Aires has the most therapists in the world!) The United Kingdom has an emphasis on cognitive behavioral therapy, other regions are more medication focused, and unfortunately probably no one will take your insurance abroad. Still, Chris had a client who did a semester of Lacanian psychoanalysis while studying in Brazil and kept up the sessions online after he got back to Boston.

Medications may be complicated abroad. Some may not be legal where you are going (stimulants and benzodiazepines being the likely ones that are restricted), or you may be held up in immigration with your prescription. One of us was held up for hours in immigration with a simple selective serotonin reuptake inhibitor (SSRI) prescription when we were lecturing in a very conservative country in the Middle East. Keep your meds in their packaging and have a doctor's note with you and check with the abroad program. Be aware that some countries or regions may not have your medication at the pharmacy, so talk with a prescriber about substitutes, or see if you can bring a semester's worth of medication. Still in other countries you might be able to just walk into a pharmacy and ask for what you need and the pharmacist can make it for you on the spot. Everywhere it will be different.

You also might think about a semester on a wilderness, service, or spiritual trip. Like going abroad, these can be life changing, and they can be challenging, too. Often these programs will want a note from your current therapist asserting that you're not a risk to yourself or others, and have a plan for how you'll manage challenges in places that might be out of cell phone or Internet range.

So we hope you do get a life-changing, or at least fun, experience doing something different. But one thing we do know is that culture shock works both ways. It can be disorienting, even triggering to go abroad or away, and it can be isolating and strange to come back home from time away when your old friends don't "get" your experience away. Plan your "re-entry" a bit with friends from your program, your supports there, and set up a soft landing for yourself as you get back home.

How Should I Disclose to Family, Friends, and Faculty/Staff About Mental Health Issues?

Whether you've been officially diagnosed or you're just aware that you're going through something, you might consider sharing that with those around you. You might do that formally by asking for accommodations as we discuss in the book, or more informally by just letting folks know. What you choose to share is largely a personal decision. Remember that not everyone will be or can be supportive of everything you might want, but hopefully at least explaining your circumstances to them will help.

Family

- *Is it safe?* Have your caregivers or other family members been supportive of you in the past? Do you know of any family members who have experienced difficulty in managing their mental health? Are any of them mental health professionals? It might be nice to have their support as you navigate sorting out your mental health while at college. The more supportive folks we have around us, the more likely we are to do well. If your caregivers or other family members make fun of mental illness, don't believe it is real, or tend to be unempathetic, it might be best to keep it to yourself. Sometimes when we find ourselves in one of those scenarios, we might want to tell them anyway, hoping that they will care or understand. However, disclosing to an unsafe person, especially someone in your family, can set off a whole other cascade of stressors and challenges—and you're already dealing with enough!

- *Who is safe and who isn't?* If it is one person, or it's everyone, share what's going on to your level of comfort. If you let them in, you let them support you. Ask for what you need, but know you might not get it. If it is more check-ins, a visit, a weekend home, or something else, see if they are able to help you meet that need. Sometimes no one feels safe, and in that case, we might rely on others who can create a community of care and support around us (friends, staff, support groups, etc.).
- *What might they need to know?* If your caregivers or other family members are involved with your health insurance, they might get a bill or explanation of benefits that you see a mental health provider or went to the hospital. In that case, they will end up finding out, so it might be best to let them know beforehand. If you are considering taking a leave of absence and intend on staying home, or have familial financial support while you're in college, they will need to know so that they can adjust as necessary.

Friends

- *Who would make for a good emotional support?* Do you have a friend who is a great listener, kind, or has dealt well with their own mental health challenges? They might make a good candidate. Allow your friend to carry some of the weight of what you're going through by sharing with them. Check in with them to see their capacity for listening before you unintentionally trauma dump.
- *Is there a way that your friends can support you?* Request something from them that might make this time more comfortable. If you've been isolating yourself, maybe ask a friend to have lunch with you on a weekly basis. Or if you want to have support from a friend who is far away, maybe schedule regular video calls. If your friend is unable to meet your need, this might feel particularly bad when you are down, but thank them for being honest and considering your request. And think of someone else who might be able to help.
- *You might want to tell some, and not tell others.* That's totally okay. This isn't some big secret that you're hiding, so don't feel guilty if you only

tell a few friends who you trust and who are supportive. This is about making you feel comfortable and reminding yourself that you have people around you who want you to be and do well. Sometimes our friends aren't the most equipped to support us through our emotional struggles, so being selective with whom you share is not unreasonable. It makes sense. It also can take time in any new friendship, romantic or platonic, to know the right time to disclose.

- *Be mindful of your material and delivery.* While you may be eager to share, sometimes our struggles make it hard to know what's appropriate to share and how. Just venting has its limits, and sometimes "dumping" our traumatic stories on others can trigger them or leave them feeling overwhelmed or helpless. It can be hard to find the balance. If you notice yourself getting overwhelmed while sharing, take a breath or sip of water, or even a moment to stretch out, so that you can recenter yourself. Chances are, the conversation is moving into territory that might be a bit intense for your friend and unhelpful for you if you are feeling that ungrounded.

Faculty and Staff

- *If it is a professor,* consider how much they really need to know. If you have a conversation with them about some late assignments, do they need to know that you haven't been able to sleep because you're having intrusive thoughts and nightmares every evening? Not really. If you say that you've been having challenges with your mental health, this should get the point across, especially if you offer a note from a mental health provider. If your professor presses you for more information around your diagnosis, medication, treatment, and so on, don't feel pressured to share it. They don't need to know that. You can politely decline and say, "I'd rather not discuss the details right now." This is where having your dean, advisor, or staff in accommodations can be helpful as they can convey the broad strokes for you so that you don't feel put on the spot by your professor. If you have a close relationship with your professor, you might feel comfortable sharing and that is okay, too. Respect their time and energy, and accept their kindness.
- *If it is a dean or advisor,* feel free to share that you're having some struggles with your mental health and that they're affecting your ability to do well. If you want to disclose your diagnosis, it is up to you, but it should not be necessary. They might need permission from you to speak to your mental health provider if you're seeing one, so you can decide if you

would like to sign off on that, or on what your mental health provider is and is not allowed to share. Usually they just write a brief note or letter at your request.

- *If it is someone working in accommodations*, you won't necessarily need to share details, but your paperwork might share them anyway. You should tell them that you need accommodations for mental health reasons at the very least, but you might want to disclose your diagnosis so that they can better support you. Chances are, they've been doing this work for a while and might know what will be most helpful, and they'll know what your college is able to provide. Further, they are the person handling your accommodations request, so keeping them in the loop is a good idea. Ideally, this person will be your ally in coming up with solutions and navigating the process.

- *You might want to tell your resident adviser (RA) or residential life staff.* Often these staff have some idea of available resources and/or some training in how to support students, so it might be helpful for you to talk to them. You shouldn't have to share any details beyond your comfort level, and be mindful of the fact that they may share information with the university if they are concerned about safety. Check the policies if you are unsure, or just ask.

- *If it is another staff member*, it is probably not necessary, but it might be something that you want to do. If there is a coach, chaplain, or another staff member whom you have a good rapport with and want support from, try telling them. Again, they may have reporting requirements and may not be able to keep everything confidential if there's a safety concern. But locating and utilizing your network of support at your college is crucial to your success. Knowing that some staff are wishing you well and wanting the best for you is helpful on those days when it feels like too much. Scheduling a check-in here and there, or getting a coffee or tea with them, might make you feel more supported.

In Conclusion

We hope that some of the wisdom from students and professionals we've shared in this chapter resonates with you and helps with the decisions you'll be making as you head to college or head back. None of this is easy, and while there are many decisions to be made, hopefully you've built a network of supportive friends, family, and professionals to help you navigate.

Chapter 3
Getting the Help You Need

Part of why we are in a mental health crisis nationally and globally is because finding help can be incredibly difficult. Not only are therapists and prescribers in short supply, but help is expensive, and insurance is incredibly complicated. Add to that stigma, logistics with timing, privacy and transportation, not to mention all the therapeutic options, and it can be easy to just give up. When you're depressed, doing anything is hard, let alone wading through bureaucracy. Anxiety can make reaching out its own challenge, neurodiversity can make prioritizing hard, and trauma and other struggles only worsen trust issues. We've also tried to offer support to those who are from more marginalized backgrounds and those for whom stigma can still feel shameful. Getting help is not easy, so hopefully you've got folks who can support you and learn from the tips in this book. We also want to demystify the therapy process a bit and offer some reality checks on what a rare hospital visit is really like.

How Do I Find a Therapist?

My depression tells me I don't have depression, just that everything sucks including me. Which also sucks, because my parents also tell me I don't have depression. Having a therapist understand, and help me find the words to talk to my parents made such a difference. I would never have graduated in the time I did without Dr. M.

—Alana, recent college graduate

While it might seem scary or overwhelming to find a therapist, the good news is, it's not as stressful as finding a date—in fact, it's easier (although there's not an app to swipe through therapists . . . yet). Almost every campus has trained therapists, and often, you can just check out the website and call or email to get more information. You can also have a friend, coach, or someone else from your support network do this for you or with you, if that makes it easier. You'd be amazed at how many students walk over to the counseling center or make the call with a friend.

If you can get a referral from someone you know that can be best because they don't just know you, but you *and* the therapist. Some of the students we've had the most successful relationships with are the ones who were sent by a dean, professor, or friend who recommended us and thought we'd make a good fit.

Toby, whom Chris saw for years as she struggled with a tough combination of depression and attention-deficit disorder (ADD), gave counseling one last shot after her writing tutor recommended him. She came to the session skeptical, but she left laughing and saying, "Thank God you weren't just another Mr. Rogers type!" And you know what? A Mr. Rogers type might be just what another student needs, and it is wonderful that they can get their needs met by a Mr. Rogers–type colleague. With about one in three college students seeking counseling these days, it's almost certain that someone you know has a recommendation of who to see (or who *not* to see). And with mental health getting more attention lately, some staff on campus (professors, deans, chaplains, etc.) may have sat through a training on mental health and know someone to recommend. Ask around!

If you don't have someone who can offer a name, you can ask your insurance company for a "behavioral health" referral or directory, or check your insurance company's online directory to see who is in network, if that's something that you need. You can also use a directory like Psychology Today or ZenCare, or just search the Internet more generally. Often you can find a little information about the mental health professional in question on their website or on an online directory that might help you make a decision about whether they could be a good fit. However, while some have extensive websites, many of our best colleagues have basically no Web presence. Still others have very impressive websites but less than impressive skills and track records. (You can't judge a book by its cover, including therapists.) If you know you want a certain kind of therapy, most specific schools of therapy have directories for those trained in their method, like dialectical behavioral therapy (DBT), for example, where you can search for someone in your area.

> It was actually my teammates from lacrosse that helped me get over to the coun-seling center when I was going through a really tough time after my girlfriend and I broke up. The team captain was actually a liaison to the mental health center, and they dragged me over to meet a campus therapist he'd met during a training he'd done.
>
> **—Tim, junior with adjustment disorder**

> Therapy was not a thing that our family did, so we were shocked at first when Alex told us he was meeting with a psychologist on campus. But some conversa-tions later about his anxiety, we were so incredibly grateful that the school covered mental health sessions as part of tuition, and know Alex is so much happier now.
>
> **—Scott, parent of a student with anxiety**

You might be surprised to learn what makes for the best psychotherapy or counseling (terms we use interchangeably in this book because they're essen-tially the same thing). The number-one factor, shown in studies over and over again, is actually not the type of therapy, or even the degree the therapist has, but the *quality of the relationship between the therapist and patient or client* (two other words we also use interchangeably). So if you feel comfortable with someone after meeting with them once or twice, stick it out. Likewise, you might wonder about the differences among psychologists, counselors, social workers, and others, but these actually matter less than your relationships and their experience. Psychiatrists and some nurses and others may provide medication, unlike the other professions, but they may also do therapy and counseling.

And when lot of people rave about their therapist, you may feel as though you should pick the perfect person. But this may be a situation where you don't need "Dr. Right"; you need "Dr. Right Now." One way that can feel easier than making a full-on commitment is, when you do reach out to set up an appointment, to ask for a few meetings for a "consultation" rather than a long-term commitment. It actually makes it easier for both of you, if it's not a good fit.

And look, if it's not a good match, we're therapists and can promise you—*we don't take it personally!* If anything, we are just happy you're getting help anywhere. (And if you do feel like your therapist has weird jealousy issues or gets possessive, that's a total red flag!)

At the same time, especially when you are depressed or anxious, *you* might take it personally if you feel like it's a mismatch or awkward at first. Even so, bring this up with your therapist. Or, if you haven't done therapy before, it might feel awkward initially, which makes sense when two strangers are forced into talking about the intimate details of one person's life. But if it feels awkward after the first few months, you might want to talk to your therapist about it to see if the situation can be rectified, or consider looking elsewhere.

Speaking of awkward, some people find that they have a bit of a crush on their therapist, and that's because it's often one of the first times we really feel seen and understood. That can take the form of wanting to be best friends with them, or even more sexual crushes, or just idealizing them. This is totally normal; in fact, therapists have a name for this: transference. It happens especially when we've felt misunderstood for so long by caregivers or our peers. Suddenly, we feel like someone gets us and that feels amazing! If you have some big feelings, you are welcome to bring these up. We therapists are used to these conversations, and they can help clear the air if it feels like your feelings are distracting from the work you're trying to do. But, no, you are not supposed to ask your therapist to hang out, even for coffee. It's nothing personal; it's just against your therapist's code of ethics and could put them at risk of losing their license and job.

Finding a therapist is a lot like Goldilocks! (Yes, the girl who committed a felony!). It felt like I had to try a few different bowls of porridge before finding the one that was just right! The first therapist I had, Ms. Carol, if she was that bowl of porridge she'd be too cold because honestly she was too old. I couldn't relate. She was always lecturing me: telling me how to think and feel. But therapy doesn't have to be like that! It can be this experience where you understand why you feel the way you feel and better understand how to manage these unpleasant emotions. Therefore, I didn't give up. I found my second therapist: Sara. Now if Sara was that bowl of porridge, she'd be too hot because she is always trying to fix me. People, especially me, don't like to be fixed. We like to feel heard. So after a few sessions, I broke up with Sara. Then, my junior year of college, I found a therapist that was just right: Erin. Erin was just right for many reasons . . . she was young . . . I could relate to her, but most importantly . . . she listened to me! I felt safe talking to Erin!

—Wes Woodson, college graduate, author, and mental health advocate

Should I Get an On-Campus or Off-Campus Therapist?

There's no two ways about it: In general, therapists are in very high demand, and on campuses, they are often in short supply. For that reason, often university counseling departments have limits on the number of sessions they can provide or strongly nudge you to get into a group or find someone off campus. In fact, we've spoken with many students who felt pushed out the door almost when they arrived, and after waiting for weeks for an appointment. After getting up the courage, that can feel like a major rejection, or invalidation, of your experience. But the demand, combined with low pay, high stress, and minimal flexibility, leads to a lot of turnover and is a systemic issue that also hits marginalized populations even harder as they may struggle to find someone whom they identify with, or something accessible.

For that reason, we suggest finding someone off campus if possible, but if you're in a bind or your college offers more extensive resources that meet your needs, try that. Either way, it's a good idea to see what your college offers in terms of counseling.

What Do I Say on a Voicemail or Email? And How Do I Get a Therapist to Call Me Back?

If you send a message or leave a voicemail, explain a little bit about who you are, what you are looking for help with, information about your insurance/finances, and your availability for a consultation and regular counseling sessions. As a therapist, the most helpful messages to get usually say something like this:

> Hi, Dr. Willard, my name is Joe College. I got your name from my roommate's mother's Pilates instructor, Tony. I'm looking for a therapist to help me with anxiety issues and hoping to set up a consult. I'm wondering if you take my insurance (insert insurance name and plan here) or know someone locally who would be a fit. You can reach me at this number at (insert best times to reach you) or email me at (insert email here.).

> Hi, Ms. Green, my name is Jeff. I'm a student at Boston University back for the semester, and I'm interviewing therapists to help me with depression. I'm hoping we could find a time to talk and see if it's a good fit with me and my insurance. I have class all day Tuesdays and Thursdays this semester but am usually around Mondays and Wednesdays.

What therapists say about getting callbacks:

> I know it shouldn't be this way, but I am more likely to call someone back if they name drop a colleague who I trust or a friend who I think of as trustworthy who sent them my way.
>
> **—Ayanna, social worker in Boston**

> When a potential client or parent tells me in a detailed way why they want to work with me, what's worked or hasn't in the past, especially if they've been to therapy before and basically show me they are motivated, that helps me call them back. Oh, and if they tell me their schedule up front, especially college kids which are always changing!
>
> **—Alan, psychologist in New Hampshire**

As a warning, not everyone will necessarily call or message you back. Don't take this personally! Unlike doctors' offices, many therapists don't have secretaries to stay on top of communication, and some therapists forget to update their listings that their practice is full. Just keep asking around, and ask if the therapists have a waiting list that you can join. It's important to reach out to as many therapists as you can to account for any availability, insurance, or other issues.

What Do I Ask in a Consultation or Phone Call?

Good news! A therapist responded to you, and you will have a consultation session or phone call. They will likely have plenty of questions for you, but there are a number of questions you might want to have for them. Below is a checklist of potential questions. Some of this might be important to you, and some less so, so decide which matter and don't hesitate to ask any of these to a potential therapist.

Finances

- Do you accept my insurance in network?
- Do you accept my insurance out of network, and if so, how does that work?
- What are your regular fees? Do you ever do a sliding scale or have payment plans for students?
- What is your policy for missed sessions or late cancellations? Do you charge for missed sessions and late cancellations?

Skills and Style

- Are you familiar with *my* mental health issues? Anxiety? Posttraumatic stress disorder (PTSD)? Depression? etc.?
- Are you familiar and/or comfortable with other aspects of who I am? (i.e., gender, sexuality, race, language, ethnicity, learning differences, medical issues, spiritual beliefs, etc.)
- Are you familiar with college students or with my school?
- Do you have a specialty? (You might want this for anxiety and depression; you will definitely want this for eating disorders, substance use, and some other conditions.)
- What type of therapy do you do? (e.g., dialectical behavior therapy [DBT], cognitive behavioral therapy [CBT], acceptance and commitment therapy [ACT], psychodynamic, etc.)
- How many years of experience do you have, and in what settings or with what populations?
- Are you an advice giver, a listener, a coach, a problem solver? How do you work?
- Do you give homework between sessions?
- Do you have a prescriber you work with?

Time Concerns

- How often do you like to have sessions and how long are they for?
- Do you do standing appointments (i.e., every Tuesday at 11a.m.), or do you schedule week by week?
- How many sessions do you think might be needed for what I described?

Other Logistics

- Do you work regularly with someone who prescribes medication?
- What's your emergency policy if I need to get in touch outside of sessions?
- Do you do telehealth or phone sessions over summers, school breaks, or other times?
- Are you easy to get to from campus?
- Do you think you can help me? If not, can you recommend someone who can?

How Do I Find a Culturally Competent Therapist?

Unfortunately, this is a really challenging issue. There is definitely an under-representation of therapists from various backgrounds in the world, and sometimes even less diverse practitioners available on campuses. Off campus may have better options, but that's probably more likely in urban areas, not in rural college towns. It's a real problem and one that the field is working hard to address, but not fast enough. We spoke with Dr. Nick Covino, the president of William James College, a psychology training school, who emphasized the urgent need to train more therapists of color and from marginalized backgrounds. Dr. Broderick Leaks, clinical associate professor in the Department of Psychiatry and the Behavioral Sciences at the Keck School of Medicine of USC and Director of the counseling center at USC Student Health, reminds us there are other folks out there (clergy, academic coaches, advisors, faculty and alumnae groups) besides clinical therapists on and near campus who can be part of your support network, too. They could serve as a mentor, friend, or casual support. (See Chapter 6 for more on building your support network.)

Dr. Charmain Jackman, a psychologist outside of Boston, addresses some of the cultural challenges as well, reminding students that campus affinity groups, centers, and houses often have staff who have some training in mental health or counseling and are often working to destigmatize mental health, and they have connections in the larger community to more diverse resources than the counseling center at school may have. Even if the affinity groups and centers don't feel like a fit for you, at least get on their mailing list or follow their socials for updates to remind yourself that you're not as alone as you might think. Pay them a visit to at least meet the program directors. You may not need it now, but it could be very helpful at a later date. You may be surprised at what these spaces can offer you.

Fortunately, we are living in a time where it is easier to find providers who match aspects of your identity, and cultural competence has become a larger part of training for folks in health care, but we certainly have a ways to go. As society continues to diversify, and we have more open conversations about intersectionality and antioppressive lenses in psychology, it can be easier to get adequate support that accounts for your background even if the person you see can't personally relate.

If you're having trouble finding a good option on campus, off-campus options may provide more variety, but that's probably more likely in urban areas, not in rural college towns. But this is a place where telehealth can shine!

Perhaps someone who is a good fit isn't in walking or driving distance, but they can see you through their chosen telehealth platform.

How Do I Even Ask About Cultural Competence?

If you are looking for a provider, it's okay to prefer someone with a similar background who is more likely to get you, just as its okay to prefer someone *not* from your background, who may not be a part of the small community you come from or may seem more objective. What matters is finding someone you feel like you can be yourself around and who you can bring up certain topics with without worrying about how you think they might feel about what you're saying. There's no shame in that. Getting support for mental health begins with feeling safe, seen, and understood. Sure, it's possible that someone from a different background or with a different set of experiences might be able to empathize, but it's totally fair for you to want someone who you feel doesn't have to translate you to understand you. Your cultural or social context is part of what you bring to the session, and you deserve to be understood.

In the event that your options are limited, or you don't mind seeing someone who might not be able to relate to your experience, we have some questions that you can ask the provider to gauge if they might be a good fit. Consider some, or all, of the following:

1. What experience do you have working with [insert identity here]?
2. What training do you have in cultural competence?
3. Generally, how diverse is your client base?
4. Are there any populations that you specialize working with?
5. What do you think about [insert systemic issue here]?
6. Are you willing to learn more about my cultural background if I share?
7. Do you speak any other languages, including mine?
8. What is your background?

We can't guarantee that they'll answer some of the more personal questions about their opinions on systemic issues or their background, but you can always ask. And when you do ask, how do you feel about their answers? If you aren't satisfied, keep looking. It's important that you feel safe and understood by your provider as much as possible. It might be difficult to find someone who is the perfect fit, but you should feel like they'll have a mostly good understanding of where you're coming from, or what your life experiences consist of, so that you feel comfortable bringing your whole self to your sessions.

How Do I Bring Up Cultural Misunderstandings With My Provider?

If you are seeing a provider who you feel does not understand a cultural element at play in your dynamic or in your life, we encourage you to bring it up. Unfortunately, we can't guarantee that they'll respond helpfully or won't get defensive, so if you don't feel like you can manage, it might be better to start looking for a better fit. Still, here's a process to try to broach the topic:

Review the situation yourself (and maybe with someone you trust)

1. What happened that made you feel uncomfortable? Is it something in general about your provider or their approach that made you feel that way? What did they not "get" or understand that you tried to share? Try to think of at least one concrete example to bring up.
2. How did that make you feel? How do you feel it impacts your relationship with them?
3. What would you like going forward? A different approach? Check in to see if they understand? Something else? Try to get clear on what it is that you need.
4. Feel free to share it with someone you trust so you can gain more clarity or even just get some empathy.

Share with your provider

1. Phew! This can be scary and overwhelming, so take some deep breaths, or do those power postures, and do something kind for yourself to gather your strength for this.
2. Decide if you'd rather bring it up during the session, perhaps at the beginning or closer toward the end (we recommend the former if you think you're going to be anxious the whole time—just do it!). If you don't feel comfortable sharing it this way, perhaps send them an email with what you want to say and say that you would like to discuss this with them. Some providers will only do this during a session, but you can also request a phone call or ask them if they can find another time to chat about it.

See if they have any questions

1. Despite all of their training, many providers can be clueless and still miss the point. See if they have any questions for you about what you said.

Take a moment to gather your feelings and thoughts

1. If you feel overwhelmed or upset by the interaction, name that with your provider. If you need some time to process, say that as well. If you completed the conversation and the feelings are hitting you after the fact, journal it out, call a friend, or try a self-care activity to settle things.

Revisit if necessary

1. If you notice that more situations are popping up that make you uncomfortable in the same vein, bring it up. If you have the capacity, bring it up as it's happening so you can point it out to your provider and have a conversation immediately. And if you feel like they are missing the point and it isn't working out, look for another provider. Someone out there can meet your needs!

Resources to Find Culturally Competent Therapists and Related Support

- Therapy for Black Girls: https://therapyforblackgirls.com/
- Black Female Therapists: https://www.blackfemaletherapists.com/
- Therapy for Black Men: https://therapyforblackmen.org/
- Black Male Therapists: https://searchblackmaletherapists.com/
- Latinx Therapy: https://latinxtherapy.com/
- Asian Mental Health Collective: https://www.asianmhc.org/
- WeRNative (for Native and Indigenous Folks): https://www.wernative.org/
- Inclusive Therapists: https://www.inclusivetherapists.com/
- National Queer and Trans Therapists of Color Network: https://nqttcn.com/en/
- The Trevor Project (for Queer Teens and Young Adults): https://www.thetrevorproject.org/
- Innopsych: Connecting Therapists of Color: innopsych.com

How Will I Pay for This?

Mental health care, like other forms of health care in the United States, is expensive. At the same time, some therapists are flexible about fees, so you can always ask if they have a "sliding scale" for students or low-income folks. You can also ask if they would waive the co-payment if you're using insurance, or if you can work out a payment plan. Don't be shy—you never know, and you won't know if you don't ask!

Also, most professionals we know *love* working with college students because they are bright, insightful, and a lot of fun even when they are struggling with challenging issues. University counseling center jobs are fiercely competitive jobs for therapists! Plus, students tend to have more flexible schedules, so therapists may be willing to slide their fee to see you early (not easy, we know) or in the middle of the day when it can be hard for them to fill their practice with 9–5 workers, or kids who are in primary or secondary school.

Many areas have local free or discount clinics to use as well, and these might be worth looking into. Colleges and universities that have degrees in clinical psychology, social work, or counseling may offer discounted therapy if you are willing to see an intern or trainee. Even some private practices have interns and trainees that can be seen at a lower rate. Websites like Open Path Collective offer a bunch of lower cost options for therapy as well.

We have created a checklist for you to review—one for using insurance and one for not using insurance, as well as a checklist with questions for your provider.

How Do I Use Insurance?

There is a lot of specific (and at times, confusing) language and terminology used by insurance companies. If you are on a caregiver's insurance, call them to ask these checklist questions, check your insurance account online, or give the insurance company a call to find out the answers.

If you are on insurance through your college, reach out to your health center or student services to get the details, or look through any emails, physical mail, or online portals where you can access your health insurance information. If you are on your own health insurance, reach out to your insurance company or look through your online portal to find the answers.

After going through everything in this section, if you're still not sure, check directly with your insurance company. The last thing you want is a hefty surprise bill. Navigating insurance can be tricky, so when in doubt, double-check.

What Do I Need to Know About Insurance?

Basic Details

- What is the name of your insurance company and plan?
- Is it a health maintenance organization (HMO) or a preferred provider organization (PPO) or point of service (POS)?

- Do I have to get a referral for mental health services from my primary care physician (PCP), or can I schedule it myself?
- Does my insurance provide coverage for in-person and/or telehealth mental health services?
- Is there an updated online portal with an in-network provider directory?

Deductibles

- Is there a deductible that needs to be met before my mental health services are covered? If so, how much is it? Has it been met for this year?

Copays and Payments

- What is my copay for individual therapy sessions? What is my copay to see a psychiatrist or a psychiatric nurse?
- What is my copay for groups, intensive outpatient programs (IOPs), or a hospitalization?
- Can you get or do you have a health service account (HSA)? (Sometimes you or your family might be given an amount of money or a debit card tax-free to spend on health care, and that includes mental health.)

Out-of-Network Benefits

- What are my out-of-network benefits for mental health?
- How do I submit a claim for out-of-network mental health services, and how long until I'm reimbursed?

Also, if your insurance (or your family's insurance) sucks, then remember that the time to pick new insurance is usually in the fall. This is called "open enrollment," and it is the time to switch, so mark your calendar ahead.

Non-Insurance

If you don't have insurance and you want to figure out what your options are, find out the answers to the below.

Non-Insurance Checklist

- Have you checked which mental health services you can get through your college's health center, and if those are free or discounted? If so, what are they? Are there any limits on services, such as duration of care or how many sessions you can receive?

- How much money can you allocate to mental health services per month?
- Can you get support from your caregivers or other family members?
- Is there a community fund or other fund at your college that can help?

What Happens in the First Session?

Typically, therapy sessions are from 45 minutes to an hour (whereas medication appointments are usually shorter after the initial evaluation, which we will touch on later). Remember that neither you nor the therapist really knows what to expect of each other. You may feel nervous, and while they might not seem nervous, remember that they are also meeting you for the first time and trying to assess if they are the best person to help you. Your job is to get your situation across to them, and their job is to help you feel comfortable enough to share so they can see if they can help. It's okay if it feels awkward.

The content of first sessions can vary. The therapist might ask you a number of basic demographic questions, run through a more formal or informal checklist, or let you share a lot about what's happening currently. They might take a lot of notes to ensure that they are getting a good grasp on you, so don't worry if there's a lot of that initially, and, yes, any notes are also confidential.

They'll usually ask about what brings you in and how long you have been facing the issue. They may ask you a bit about your family and growing up, or if you or anyone in your family has any other mental health or medical issues. There may be uncomfortable questions about things like trauma, self-harm, suicide, and homicide. They might also ask what is going well and your strengths, as well as inquiring about challenges. While there will likely be some difficult questions in there, you don't necessarily have to answer or go into detail right away.

In the first meeting, your therapist should also review things like confidentiality, payment, insurance, and other policies to get on the same page if you didn't already go over those in a consultation or phone call prior to the visit. Feel free to ask your questions at any time, or ask for a reminder if you forget.

Dr. John Sommers-Flanagan shared a bit about how clients can get the most out of sessions, too. He said to be as open and authentic as possible, and just get out what's been on your mind recently. Remember, the therapist can't help you unless they really know what's going on. If you are nervous about sharing darker thoughts, you can always ask again about confidentiality. But, remember, their job is to be as nonjudgmental as possible, and they've probably seen and heard a lot.

Still, if you're uncertain about trust, try just sharing a bit in the first session and see how the therapist reacts. If you feel safe, keep going, and allow the trust to build. But remember, even in graduate school, they don't teach us how to read minds. We can only do what we can with the information you let us in on.

Do you have something you want to bring up? You're allowed to ask questions, push back, express what you feel like is working or not, and ask for what you need. After all, you're the paying customer and should be getting the services you want and need!

And lastly, sometimes, once you connect with a therapist, they might share that they aren't the right person to support you, and that they're not able to work with you. That doesn't mean you are helpless or hopeless, but just that there is someone who will be a better fit. A good therapist will be honest about this and give you a list of names because different people just have different skill sets, and there *is* someone out there who can better help you!

I went to the university counseling center after a breakup. I felt really stupid because it was just a breakup, but I was losing sleep and couldn't eat anything and my RA [resident advisor] told me to go. The counselor was super nice, and just asked me some questions about myself, and let me know I wasn't wasting his time like I worried. We only needed to meet three times, but it was super helpful.
—**Charlotte, first-year student dealing with adjustment issues and anxiety**

I was not sure about seeing someone because my faith is important to me. I was worried that a counselor would judge me based on my beliefs when I was far from home in a less religious part of the country. I don't think the person I met had the same background, but it didn't matter anyway; they respected it that my faith was central to my life and to my getting better again and also gave me some cool tools and tricks to manage my mood better.
—**Chrystal, junior dealing with depression**

My parents sent me as a kid when they were getting divorced and all I remember was that we played checkers and I got a root beer at the end, and I didn't get the point it felt like a waste of my time. . . . I didn't know what to expect as an adult, except no root beer! But it was really different, I mean, obviously, but it felt like my space, and I was able to use therapy in a really different way. It makes such a difference when you are grown up and want to go on your own.
—**Matt, sophomore dealing with social anxiety**

What Your Therapist Might Recommend After the First Session

"You should join a group." Groups are a great way to meet other folks you can relate to who are working on similar issues. They might be to learn skills, like DBT groups, identity-related (i.e., for students of color), or for a certain diagnosis or issue.

"You should see an expert or specialist in this issue." Some general therapists might think you'd be better served by someone with certain expertise if they don't specialize in that area, or are unable to handle more complex situations (i.e., dual diagnoses, substance use, obsessive-compulsive disorder [OCD] or disordered eating). But in general, most therapists are pretty qualified to handle anxiety, depression, trauma, and other more common concerns.

"You should try a certain kind of therapy." Similar to the last point, perhaps your therapist thinks you would benefit from seeing someone who specializes in a certain therapy and will make that recommendation to you.

"You should try medication." Sometimes things are so intense that finding a medication could help more immediately. Usually it's not at a first session that you'll hear this, but it can happen (and we share more on medication on Chapter 5).

"You might want to get tested, evaluated, or screened." When therapists want more information and are unable to get it with their skill set or training, they might recommend that you get a screening or psychological testing. Again, this is not usually after session one, but you never know. These can be very brief and just a few questions, or they can be more extensive. Different psychological testing can tell you a lot about your learning style and personality, assess you for conditions like attention-deficit/hyperactivity disorder (ADHD) or autism spectrum disorder (ASD), get clarity around which accommodations that are needed, and/or generally help you understand yourself better.

"You should go to the hospital." More on this later, but this is extremely rare in the first meeting.

"Let's keep working together if you'd like, and let's see if we can do good work together." This is the most common, and probably also the most relieving, recommendation you'll hear.

What Is Confidentiality? What Would I Have to Say or Do to Cause My Therapist to Break Confidentiality?

Seeing a therapist might feel like you're journaling out loud. And it's true; you might feel a great sense of relief having a person and place where you can freely unload. However, unlike a journal, this is a person, and you don't want just anyone to have access to your innermost thoughts, and it isn't necessarily totally private. For this reason, ask your therapist for specifics on confidentiality. While there are general guidelines that all must follow, these can vary somewhat from provider to provider. Ask about which specific instances would lead them to breaking confidentiality, and feel free to ask them to provide examples as well to make sure that you understand. And if you have any specific curiosities, just ask. "Would you send me to the hospital if I said xyz?" "Would you call the police if I said that xyz?" And you may be surprised to know that even illegal things like doing drugs or robbing a bank will not result in your therapist breaking confidentiality. Again, please ask your therapist, as this can vary, but generally, the following might lead to a break in confidentiality: plans or serious intent to harm oneself; plans or serious intent to harm another person (this doesn't apply to those with OCD); any mentions of child, elder, or dependent abuse; a judge's court order; and local laws in your area.

What Do I Need to Know About Suicide?

Of all the serious mental health concerns in this book, none is more concerning than suicide. In 2023, 25% of college students reported having passing thoughts about suicide, with 10% even moving forward with creating a plan. In the 12 months prior to the survey, 3% of students reported attempts.[1] And whether in college or not, suicide is a major component of the mental health crisis across the nation.[2]

Suicidal thoughts and behavior exist on a continuum. On the one end, a student might more passively wish that they were dead, or think, "If the car crashed, I wouldn't care." Others might actively be planning or exploring options. Some may even acquire the means, and others may go all the way to act on their suicide plan. Anywhere on the spectrum is concerning and worth seeking professional help. If you've planned out or acted on a suicidal urge, it is critical to get to emergency services as soon as possible. But even if you "only" have thoughts of death or suicide, reach out soon as you can, because most suicidal actions start with thoughts.

And even though it may be hard to imagine, with the right treatment and support, people can overcome suicidal thoughts and behaviors. Millions of people have.

What Are the Signs of Suicidal Thinking?

If you experience any of the following, or see them in another, you should consider reaching out for help. It stands to reason that any thinking or talking about, or acting on, suicidal thoughts is the clearest indication, but there are others:

- Posting more ambiguous or passively suicidal thoughts on social media
- Researching suicide online
- Feeling trapped, as though the pain is unbearable
- Feeling like a burden to others
- Feeling like the world would be better off without you
- Thinking others would not care much if you were gone
- Thinking about, talking about, or posting online any suicide or violent theme
- Giving away important possessions
- Suddenly feeling light after feeling very heavy

The bottom line is this: If you or someone you know is experiencing any of the above, never ignore these and get help immediately. And if it is someone else, know that asking someone if they are suicidal will not plant the idea in their head (despite the myths out there). Remember that the vast majority of people can feel better, and so can you.

What Do I Do If I or Someone Else Is Suicidal?

If you or someone you know is suicidal, you can get immediate help by dialing 988, which is the Suicide and Crisis Lifeline, or access their online chat at https://988lifeline.org/chat. They will connect you to local resources for help. You can also call 911, or the campus police or psychological service crisis line. If you are with someone who is suicidal, stay with them until help arrives and keep them in your sight.

How Honest Can I Really Be With My Therapist? I Don't Want to End Up in the Hospital!

A common worry among clients in the first few sessions is whether we will send them to the hospital. Given that hospitalization, particularly when it is against one's will, can be traumatizing, we aren't interested in sending a client there unless there is a real and imminent danger. It is not abnormal to feel hopeless, withdrawn, and exhausted with your life circumstances. We understand that and encourage our clients to be honest about that so that we can try to come up collaboratively with a plan to get you the level of support you need.

Talking about thoughts you are having is very different than telling a therapist you have a specific plan to kill yourself that afternoon, and we understand that and act accordingly. As Dr. Sommers-Flanagan reminds us, thinking about death is far more likely a sign of psychological pain than it is a sign that you are actually a risk to yourself. Also OCD-like fears and thoughts that you might hurt yourself or someone else will not lead to hospitalization!

Why Would Anyone Go to the Hospital?

The vast majority of students who struggle with mental illness will never need to go to the hospital for treatment. But sometimes the level of pain and hopelessness is more than you can handle alone. A hospital or inpatient program may be the best place to feel safe, kickstart therapy, or adjust your medications. Most hospital stays are short, because the goal is to use the time to get you back into your life as quickly as possible.

The most common reasons students might need a hospital stay have to do with your ability to cope safely with your mental illness symptoms on campus. Typically, this happens in the following situations:

1. Deciding yourself you need a higher level of care
2. Presenting a significant risk to self or others, including a plan for suicide or a suicide attempt
3. Having hallucinations or other psychotic symptoms that can make you a danger to yourself or others
4. Experiencing a bad reaction to or dependence on substances
5. Having a significant eating disorder that requires immediate medical intervention

How Do I Get Into the Hospital?

Once you have decided to go to the hospital, or someone else has, you just go to the nearest regular hospital or one with a relationship to your school · if there's not a mental hospital nearby. If you are considered safe and not an immediate danger to yourself or someone else, you might go with a friend or family member, or even take a taxi or rideshare. If you are considered an immediate danger, or are unable to make decisions for yourself, you might be transported by ambulance. That can be scary, and sometimes campus security might also be around, but usually they are trained to be supportive and stay out of the way.

Depending on the circumstances, you will either be admitted directly to the psychiatric unit, or you may have to wait. We have seen a huge increase in demand for beds in recent years, and in some parts of the country, you may have to wait in the emergency department for hours or even days. This in and of itself can be stressful. If you're choosing to go, you should have time to pack your toiletries, change of clothes, books, and phone charger, but in some cases, if it is an emergency, you may have to have a trusted roommate, friend, or family member bring these for you, after you have been admitted.

One thing to know is that there are many things that hospital units either won't allow you to bring or won't allow you to keep with you while you are there; these items will be kept locked up safe by staff. Typically, those are things that could harm you or others that seem more obvious, like medications (including over-the-counter substances), as well as drugs and alcohol.

Once You Are Officially Admitted

There are likely going to be many interviews with a variety of intake people, many of whom you won't see again, and then some with the mental health experts who will work with you during your stay. It can be very frustrating answering the same questions over and over again; however, know that often each person is asking from a different point of view, and it is for your benefit. For instance, if you are feeling suicidal, the insurance person may be asking so that they can get certain days authorized by your insurance carrier, the nurse may be asking to see if you need close monitoring, the psychiatrist may be asking because they need to determine what medication you should be taking, the case manager may be asking to help determine aftercare, the therapist might be asking to see if there are skills that you need help with in your current situation, and so on.

What Happens in the Hospital?

In hospital, you can be in close contact with therapists and nurses, get medications right away (if you need medication), and access treatments you can't get at home. The purpose of going to the hospital in a crisis is so experts can keep an eye on you in order to keep you safe, determine what extra help you might need, and give you some rest from the demands of school. Once you are feeling better and ready to go home, case managers can help you set up outpatient appointments and your doctors can be in touch with your home psychiatrist to discuss medication changes. They might recommend switching up therapists and treatment teams on the outside as well.

In most hospitals, the stays are very short; for example, if you are hearing voices, the doctors might increase the medication until you are no longer hallucinating and then send you back home. In other hospitals, there are skills groups that can teach you some behavioral and meditation skills and other tools for a week or two. It depends on your case. For better or for worse, staff members are often under pressure to send you home quickly due to financial and insurance reasons. Despite recent laws mandating equal treatment for mental and medical health, it can still be prohibitively expensive, or your insurance may refuse to pay beyond a certain amount of time regardless of your mental health professional's opinion.

Although there are many benefits to being in the hospital, some students feel infantilized. Just as you get all the freedom you could want on campus, now you are faced with restrictions like bedtimes and other limitations. Often you don't get to keep your phone, and if you are at risk for suicide, you don't get to keep your shoelaces or belts, and your personal toiletries such as shampoos and razors are kept in the nursing office. The staff is focused on keeping you safe and others on the unit safe, so your freedoms might be limited to do so.

Another real thing that is *not* great about the hospital system for mental health is the journey often starts with everyone in the same place. Maybe you are depressed, in which case it can be overwhelming, if not scary, to see someone in there who is having hallucinations or threatening to act violently. Or maybe you are struggling with substances, and it can be a surprise to be rooming with someone who just tried to kill themself. Or maybe everyone else seems like they are doing fine, and you are the only one struggling. You are also likely to be in there with people of all ages, especially at first. You might feel different from everyone else on the unit, but some helpful advice is to try to identify, not compare, with other people's experiences. That's one of the mantras many students have told us have been helpful in the hospital.

Still, the vast majority of our patients are glad that they went, despite all the negatives we have just mentioned, and many students actually like their stay in the hospital. It can feel like time flies because they are so intense and jam-packed with groups, sessions, treatments, and the like, kind of like the intensity you experience when you go to camp or even college. You can even get close to a new group of people you never imagined you would be close to. It can be so validating to be with others going through similar struggles, and you might leave with not just better mental health and coping skills, but good friends.

Almost everyone we've ever met who works or has worked on inpatient units in hospitals is dedicated, competent, and compassionate. Remember, though, that these mental health professionals are human beings with stressful jobs and, like all humans, aren't perfect. Whereas in other eras, patients were frequently strapped down in restraints and administered medication against their will, the days of the overuse of involuntary restraints and sedation are over. And you don't need to worry about being kept in the hospital forever. In fact, they can only legally keep you involuntarily for three or four days (depending on which state you're living in), at which point the hospital must discharge you or petition a court that you are at such risk to yourself and/or others that you must be kept involuntarily. Even in these circumstances, the hospital has to give you access to a lawyer or the patient's rights office. And remember, when you depart, that's the highest-risk time, so make a good aftercare plan for yourself, and don't leave until you have one in place.

It was overwhelming, but honestly, everyone was so nice, the time went by really fast, and it felt like I was back at school in no time. I mean, I didn't love it, but I met some cool people, some kids that had some really bad problems, and I think I learned some good things in the groups.

   —Mark, a freshman who had just been diagnosed with depression

I was surprised by how much I liked the people. The one thing that surprised me the most was everyone's amazing dark humor—I've literally never laughed so much in my life. Even the staff who weren't therapists, in general they were easier to talk to on the floor than some of the actual therapists. My advice is to get to know those staff, they're the ones who are really good listeners, at least where I went.

   —Marisa, a college junior who went to the hospital after a suicide attempt

I actually wanted to go. I couldn't deal at all with school, my parents, and my friends. It was hard to go back to the real world, but the staff had been in touch with my parents and people at school, and the professors didn't know what happened, but I got extensions on all my work and so that was all taken care of.

—Kristin, a college junior with depression and borderline personality disorder

Olivia did not want to go, and we didn't want her to go either; the school actually sent her to the hospital and that was the worst phone call I'd ever received in my life. She didn't want to go before she went; she was so upset about being there at first, but she was definitely glad that she went in retrospect and a little scared to leave. They stabilized her and started her on medication, which was so important. It certainly didn't fix everything, but it was the beginning of a long journey that we're still in as a family, but we are far from where we started.

—Jen, mother of a college sophomore hospitalized after a psychotic episode

What Happens After the Hospital? (Aftercare)

After a few days in the hospital, once you are feeling that your life is in more control, that the symptoms are less intense, and/or that your medications have been adjusted, the goal is to discharge you. You might be sent to an intensive program (described below), or sent back to school or home with the right medications or referrals for a therapist (if you don't already have one).

Ideally, you are well enough to return to school, but you may need to take a leave of absence. Your school may also want you to be cleared medically or psychiatrically to return, and you may even have to talk to the university staff or college counselors to make your case to come back.

What Are the Intensive Programs That I Might Be Sent To?

For some students, being back in outpatient care is not enough even if they don't need a full inpatient stay. For those students, there are intermediate options between inpatient and outpatient care. These are some of the options, from least restrictive to most restrictive:

- **Intensive outpatient program (IOP)**: This is usually a few days a week for a few hours a day.
- **Partial hospitalization program (PHP) or "day treatment"**: This is a five-day-a-week program six to eight hours per day. The schedule and resources are like the hospital, but typically you sleep at home or at your dorm.

- **Community integration program, supportive living, or halfway house**: An unlocked, less intensive "therapeutic environment" where you live with other folks getting back on their feet. There are some staff who come in occasionally, and you generally have more freedom. Typically no guests and no substances are allowed, and often there's a curfew.

How Do I Manage Cultural and Family Barriers to Treatment?

Depending on your background, seeking treatment might not just be discouraged but stigmatized or deemed a betrayal. Getting support for your mental health issues might bring up judgment, confusion, or laughter from your community or family, leading to shame, undermining, or outright sabotage. Considering how many college students look to caregivers for financial and emotional support, or might be on their insurance, this can cause issues if your caregivers are skeptical or fearful of you getting support.

Before you even start to sort out your options in terms of seeking treatment, see if you can find an identity-based group or center on campus to connect with others from your community. If your campus doesn't have one, see if you can find one online or in the area.

If your school can provide treatment without getting caregivers involved, that may be the easiest and safest option for you. Let the counseling center staff know that it is a delicate situation due to your background and that you might not have support from your family and see what options are available; this won't be the first time they've helped someone through this.

If you are on your caregivers' insurance and are worried that they might get a notification, you might hesitate. What's worse: telling them beforehand, or having them find out on their own? Neither sounds great. But if you have no other option, you might have to take the risk. Even if they don't agree, your mental health is important, and we've never met a student who regretted prioritizing their mental health, even if it creates discomfort back at home.

This is another reason why it's so important to find others with similar struggles. It can be so isolating and embarrassing when other students are more open and get more support. You might feel like the odd one out, or feel upset when you see how easily a friend gets emotional support from their parents. Lean on your support network and seek connection, whether it be an affinity group on campus, your team, a support group, your friends, your therapist, or anywhere.

How to Broach the Conversation With Your Caregivers

Prepare

- What is it that you need to say? What do you need to get out of this conversation? What do you want from them? Write out a draft to get a better idea of what it is that you're trying to share.
- Now that you have some clarity about what you want to share, refine your points and do some research. Do you need to share details about a specific treatment, such as what it is, how long it lasts, or how much it costs? Would it help to educate them or offer resources about mental health so that they understand better?
- Which approach is best for your audience? Should you print out your information and hand it out, make a PowerPoint presentation, send them an email or write them a letter, or just sit together and have a conversation? Prepare accordingly.
- If you have a friend or sibling, or another support, ask for help with the process, to read what you wrote, role-play, or be with you.

Share your information

- Go through the process of sharing, whether it is sending that email or going through with a full-blown presentation. If you need paper or notes on your phone, go for it. There is no shame in needing a reminder.

Gauge their openness as concretely as possible

- Now that you've spoken your truth, ask if they have any questions. Do your best to answer them, or if you don't know the answer, tell them you will get back to them.
- Ask if they're willing to help. If it's financially, how much can they contribute? If it's emotionally, ask for what you need, which may include space and time. If it's with looking into options, ask them when they are available to chat or research options together.

Give yourself some aftercare

- How did it go? We hope that it went well and you can feel some relief. But if it didn't, do at least one kind thing for yourself. Maybe call a friend to vent, write in your journal, go for a run, or find something funny or light to watch. It's hard to share and face this kind of rejection, especially from your caregivers, so if you are feeling down, we hope that you can see how brave you just were.

Take your next steps

- Are they open to helping? Follow up on that. If not, explore the options you do have that don't include them.

This may be hard, and not seem worth it, and we get that. We want you to feel safe. It's hard enough to work through your mental health challenges as it is, and if you do think it will make it worse, wait and exhaust your other options first.

How Do I Get Privacy for Telehealth?

If you feel comfortable, explain to your roommate that you need some weekly time for therapy or a private meeting. If they push for more information, just say that you aren't able to talk about it. College is weird. It's one time in your life when you might be forced to be in a small space with one or more random people who you might never be near otherwise. This is the situation you and your roommate(s) are stuck with, so you're just trying to make it work for you. Don't feel guilty about asking for what you need!

If you can't work it out with your roommate, does a friend or your RA have space they can offer? Can you sit in your or a friend's car? What other space is there on campus—get creative. Book a private study carrel, classroom, or rehearsal space, or ask your counseling center if they know of any private spaces on campus. Maybe there is even a quiet area outside where you make your calls.

What Is Psychological Testing or Neuropsychological Testing?

One of the recommendations you may get is to seek out testing—psychological testing or neuropsychological testing—or an evaluation of some kind. Neuropsychological testing might sound interesting, or it might sound intimidating, but it can be really helpful to understand how you learn and perceive the world. These kinds of tests can be incredibly useful, but they are time consuming and often expensive. That said, insurance sometimes covers them, and sometimes universities have testing or screening centers for cheap or free. As always, it never hurts to ask!

Testing is usually recommended if you are having academic struggles, to check for executive functioning or learning issues, screen for autism, or help you get to know your learning style. They may also help clarify the root cause of what you're dealing with. For example, whether a struggle to focus is about anxiety or ADHD, or a struggle to read is depression or dyslexia.

If things aren't going well, especially academically, there may be something that's been undiagnosed. Tina Bryson reminds us that often smart, high-functioning students also hit a limit in college, especially when mental health issues strike, and those demands begin to max out their capacity for social and academic demands. When this happens, it's a great moment to investigate if there is something more to the story. Maybe there's a learning difference beneath the surface, or perhaps it is ADHD or mild autism that was missed because you've been such a good student until the most recent struggles in school. (This is particularly true for young women.)

The feedback session with the tester can help you and your support network better understand how you view the world, and get a chance to think through the types of school, classes, accommodations, and even what kinds of jobs would be a good fit for your learning style and brain.

You might sometimes be recommended to other psychological tests like the Rorschach, (yeah, the inkblot one), or extensive computer personality tests like the Minnesota Multiphasic Personality Inventory (MMPI). You may also need to complete a risk evaluation to go back to school, or a substance abuse assessment. Any of these might feel punitive, and you might be tempted to game the system, but please just be honest. This will help you get the support you need going forward. Trying to game the system will only set you back, and the tests are designed to screen for people lying. Show up, engage fully, and allow yourself to be supported.

To be clear, none of these tests works like an x-ray that will perfectly reveal your exact personality and issues. In fact, one of us, we won't mention names, got in trouble in graduate school for referring to the Rorschach as modern-day tea leaf readings. But still, they can help you learn about some blind spots you didn't know about yourself, or validate worries you've had or those around you have had. Moreover, if a diagnosis does come up, you've now got something official to bring to the accommodations or disabilities office, which we discuss in Chapter 1.

In Conclusion

We hope we've been able to help you simplify the process of getting help, as well as understand and demystify the start of the therapeutic journey, navigate some of the barriers to treatment, and figure out how to access the resources you'll need for your mental health journey.

Chapter 4
What Kind of Therapy Do I Need?

Now that you have decided that therapy is right for you, the next question is what kind of therapy do you need? Therapists joke a lot about the "alphabet soup" of therapies out there. CBT, DBT, ACT, AEDP, MBT, TFP, IFS, and many, many others. You should know that the two best predictors of whether therapy will work for you are these: (1) Does the therapy match your needs? (2) Is your therapist a good fit for you? Still, you might want to know what you're getting into, and this section will help you understand a bit about what to expect with the most common types of therapies. This list of types of therapies is not exhaustive but covers a wide range of approaches. Another question people ask is, What's the difference between therapy, psychotherapy, and counseling? For the purposes of this section, we'll use these terms interchangeably.

What Is Psychodynamic or Psychoanalytic Therapy?

Psychoanalytic psychotherapy, the type popularized by Dr. Sigmund Freud, is the original and oldest of all therapies. Even though it's often considered out of date, along with some highly questionable gender politics, it is still practiced today. The best known descendent of psychoanalysis is what we now call psychodynamic therapy (PDT), and it addresses the way that our earliest relationships, childhood and family dynamics, contribute to our struggles today. It explores the ways that these early attachments impacted your mental health, as well as your ongoing behaviors and patterns, and it can be really helpful for self-understanding. PDT is probably the closest to what you think of when you imagine psychotherapy or counseling of some kind.

What Is Cognitive Behavioral Therapy?

Cognitive behavioral therapy (CBT) was developed by Dr. Aaron Beck in the 1960s, and it challenged many of the principles of psychoanalysis. It was considered revolutionary at the time, and it is the best researched of all the therapies. The fundamental principle is that thoughts and behaviors are what make us happy and bring us fulfillment, and so when we change our thoughts and behaviors, we feel better. Beck's CBT also recognizes that many of our unhappy thoughts are due to "thinking errors," or "stinkin' thinkin'," more formally called "cognitive distortions,"[1] which we list below. These are helpful to identify in yourself, especially as they relate to anxiety and depression.

What Are Cognitive Distortions?

All-or-Nothing/Black-or-White Thinking
Black-and-white thinking is an all-or-nothing approach—deciding that things are either all bad or all good, rather than seeing them as shades of gray and as complicated as they are.

> Declan was somewhere between shy and anxious. He was excited to go out to the bars with a group of friends from his hall, because people had told him that in college he needed to "put himself out there" to make friends. But as soon as he got to the first bar, he started to feel anxious about all the people he didn't know and worrying about his ID getting rejected at the bar. Rather than remembering that there would be some stressful or awkward moments and some fun ones throughout the night, he decided he hated the whole bar scene and hated everyone who liked it, ended up clinging to one friend, then said he felt sick before leaving early and felt embarrassed about that.

Are there times you've noticed yourself or others falling into black-and-white thinking?

Discounting the Positive

This thought distortion involves looking at events through a negative lens only and disregarding the positive. The result is a pessimistic, anxious view of the world.

> After Miguel got into his top school, he spent more and more time in group chats with other admitted students. But after some interactions with others, before long, Miguel started psyching himself out, feeling like a fraud, and thinking the only reason he'd gotten in was a mistake, or just because of diversity. He had been studying hard all through high school, but rather than seeing what he had done to contribute to his own success, he decided that his success was due to chance or pity. By the time he got to campus in the fall, he'd basically logged out of the chat and was so anxious he didn't want to talk to anyone else, thinking they'd also know he was an admissions error. This really set him back socially, and he struggled to make friends through his first year.

Have there been times when you discounted the positive and only looked at the negative reasons why something good happened? Write down the ways in which you discount positive events and focus only on the negative.

Catastrophizing

Catastrophizing means seeing everything as a disaster or making sweeping negative conclusions based on minimal evidence.

> Natalia had ongoing stomach issues and started to worry about it. Pretty soon she was completely freaking out, telling everyone she knew, unable to sleep, and convinced that she had some kind of food allergy, or maybe even stomach cancer. Or could she be pregnant? The more she read about it online, the worse she felt, as she fell into a rabbithole of doom and gloom online. By the time she saw a doctor, she was convinced she had only a few months to live and had cut many foods out of her diet. But it turned out she had irritable bowel syndrome, a common health issue for people with anxiety, and that worsens with more anxiety and stress. Soon she was treating her anxiety with CBT and mindfulness, and her stomachaches faded.

What does catastrophizing look like in your life? Are there certain areas or themes that you tend to engage in catastrophizing more often? Why?

Emotional Reasoning

Emotional reasoning is coming to conclusions based on your present mood state. For instance, if you are sad, you might conclude that your romantic partner is leaving you; if you are jealous, you might conclude that they are seeing someone else; if you are happy, you might conclude that they are going to propose marriage. In the heat of the moment, when we are particularly hungry, activated emotionally, lonely, tired, or stressed (HALTS), our brains fail to think clearly and rationally. Something feels real, and so we believe that it must be real and will be real.

> Jake, a sophomore soccer recruit, always felt wiped out after a test, partly because he had so much nervous energy and had often not gotten enough sleep. Not surprisingly, he walked out of every exam feeling terrible, assumed he must have failed, and yet his grades were fine. It was starting to impact his friends and family, who would roll their eyes and not even ask about school. When he talked to his RA [resident advisor], he realized that feeling terrible after a test did not mean that his performance actually was terrible. His RA had been to therapy herself, and reminded Jake "feelings aren't facts," which became his mantra.

Do you come to conclusions based on your emotional state? If so, what are some examples? What conclusions do you think you would come to if you were in a different mood state?

Perfectionism

Some college students struggle with perfectionism, which is a striving for flawlessness together with setting exceedingly high standards for performance. It becomes a mental health issue when it is associated with the tendency to be overly critical when they fail, and then fearing failure, which leads to the tendency to procrastinate.

> Emi, a senior applying to law schools, felt like she had to be the best athlete, best student, and most beautiful or it was not worth trying. Because she set her expectations so high, there was never a chance she would actually meet them. This left her forever disappointed in herself and anxious about everything. She worked together with her therapist and her youth rabbi from home to set realistic, internal, and personal goals for success, rather than measuring herself against others all the time. Practicing self-compassion (see more about this on Chapter 6), she was able to see that all she ever knew about how perfect anyone else was what they showed the world on social media or bragged about in the dorm. She loved the slogan "Don't compare your insides to other peoples' outsides."

Do you recognize signs of perfectionism in yourself? Reflect in your journal about what you notice.

Mind Reading

Mind reading has two elements. The first is the problematic aspect, which happens when you assume to know what someone else is thinking without having much to go on. The second is a healthier version when you can accurately and empathically read nonverbal clues to understand another person's experience.

> Kobe would jump to conclusions, especially when they were stressed. Whenever their roommate Paul was quiet, they'd just assume Paul was mad at them about something and start feeling guilty and apologizing for things like not being neater in the room. When Paul insisted he was just stressed about his own exams, Kobe would then start to assume that Paul was annoyed at them for making it awkward. The cycle continued, and Kobe felt like they were walking on eggshells, even though Paul didn't actually care.

We all do mind reading to some extent. Write down the times you have been accurate and the times that you've made negative assumptions on the basis of little information. Reflect on what this shows you about your tendency to mind read.

Mental Filtering

Mental filtering is a type of cognitive distortion in which a person focuses only on the negative elements of a situation and filters out the positive ones.

> Keisha spent hours getting her outfit ready with friends, all of whom were so excited about what they were wearing to the formal. When she got to dinner, her boyfriend's friend made a comment about her jacket. Instead of recognizing that her other friends, but most importantly she herself, liked her outfit, she immediately worried that she had committed a fashion faux pas. She started feeling self-conscious and ended up carrying her coat to the party, refusing to wear it. She spent the night worried that her friends and her boyfriend thought her jacket was weird, and couldn't focus on the positive comments she was getting on not only her outfit but also her hair and nails. She was so anxious that she ended up drinking too much and woke up the next day even more embarrassed. She had filtered out the positive and focused only on the perceived negative of the situation.

Write down some instances where you have filtered out the positive and then consider how you might be able to pause and focus on the positive moving forward.

Personalizing

Personalizing is the distortion where you might attribute the entire blame for an event or situation on yourself, even when there is little to no evidence that you are to blame. It is a way of discounting external factors, ones that you have little control over, but imagine that you do.

> When Paolo, a first-generation pre-med major, was struggling with his physics problem set, he reached out to the TA [teaching assistant], who didn't respond. Paolo's immediate assumption was that the TA didn't like him, or that the TA thought Paolo's case was hopeless and that he didn't care. Paolo made the TA's response about himself, and he did so in the absence of knowing about the TA's reasons. Paolo's roommate pointed out that he was making assumptions and personalizing the situation and that there may be many reasons why the TA had not responded—for instance, he may have had his own finals, too, or had something else going on—and encouraged him to reach out to the TA again.

Can you think of a situation where something happened, and you made it all about you and how you are to blame? How was this situation impacted by external factors, or things that you don't have control over?

Shoulding and Musterbation

CBT therapists like to joke about these two puns, which are basically dad jokes. (By the way, have you ever noticed how not funny most therapists are?) The point is to always watch out for the words you use or the words of others who are struggling.

"Should" and *"must."* "I should be doing better," "I should be making more friends," "I should be dating this person or that person," "I should have gotten into that other school." "Must" statements include "I must always get As" or "I must get that internship if I want to get into grad school." There are a lot of other red-flag words that we look for in conversations as well, listening carefully to the words in our own head, and that we and others say out loud. Here are a few of the more dangerous ones: *all, always, every, everyone, everything, every time, have to, need to, must, never, no one.* In a workshop we did on campus, the resident advisors and peer leaders we worked with often found it helpful to learn about these warning words.

What Else Do I Need to Know About CBT?

We've shared a partial list of cognitive distortions, but there are many more. Remember, you don't have to have mental illness to fall into these thinking traps. Everyone makes them; however, when they significantly start to impact various aspects of your college life, they become a problem that needs addressing.

And remember, too, that these distortions are made worse by stress. They are worse if you're hungry, lonely, tired, and sleep deprived. They can be triggered by certain people, places, and things. They are made worse by trauma and societal judgments, all of which set the stage for internalizing a negative sense of self.

CBT helps to reframe these issues, add more evidence or context to see the big picture, and correct the errors. Sometimes mindfulness, breathing, or progressive relaxation is a part of CBT as well, since these relax the body and brain, opening it up to new perspectives that we can't access when we are overwhelmed. Of course, we have to recognize our thoughts before we can change them, so CBT includes tools like thought logs, rating your mood and behavioral symptoms, and uses scales from 1 to 10 in different situations to rate these.

CBT is the treatment with the best evidence base for anxiety and depression. It focuses less on exploring your past and more on changing what can be changed by taking new, more accurate perspectives on your thoughts and perceptions about yourself, the world, and the future.

What Is Dialectical Behavior Therapy?

Dialectical behavior therapy (DBT) is a type of talk therapy that was developed to help manage overwhelming emotions. [2] Emotions can be so powerful and painful that in some people they can trigger suicidal thoughts, self-injury, substance misuse, and other destructive behaviors. DBT was developed by Dr. Marsha Linehan (1993),[3] a psychologist at the University of Washington, who not only was inspired by mindfulness but found that psychodynamic and cognitive behavioral therapies were not enough.

The word *dialectical* in DBT means that there can be different perspectives on any situation, and someone can learn to integrate or synthesize truths, even if they seem to be polar opposites. Basically it means being able to hold and tolerate two different perspectives at once—a mark of emotional intelligence.

For example, for those with intense emotions, self-harm works to reduce the suffering. Of course, it also creates problems. In this situation what an outsider sees as a problem (or one truth) is actually seen as a solution (another truth) to the person self-harming. How can we hold these seemingly opposite ideas when they seem contradictory? The solution of cutting, which is effective in the short term yet problematic in the long term, is one answer to the problem of intense and painful emotions. When both the person suffering and the people in their lives can recognize this, they have moved toward a new understanding of the behavior.

Dialectics is about combining opposite ideas into a new idea. Opposites abound in DBT, including integrating Eastern philosophy and acceptance strategies with Western change techniques derived from CBT. The most fundamental of these seemingly opposite truths are that in order to help someone change, we must first accept the person as they are. Linehan was not the first to acknowledge this. As a humanistic psychologist Carl Rogers put it, "only by accepting myself as I am, can I begin to change."

Change is integrated with acceptance. At the individual level, DBT focuses on helping people accept the reality of their lives and their behaviors as a launching point for them to learn the skills necessary to change their lives, by not only increasing helpful behaviors but also reducing their unhelpful behaviors.

What Type of Issues Is DBT Useful For?

Many people who benefit from DBT recognize that they are emotionally sensitive. They tend to feel things more deeply than others and more quickly than others, and when they have an emotional reaction, it tends to take them longer to settle back down to their emotional baseline. They might even identify as highly sensitive people (HSPs).

DBT has proven to be effective for treating and managing a wide range of mental health conditions, including borderline personality disorder, self-injury, posttraumatic stress disorder (PTSD), eating disorders, and anxiety disorders, as well as addictions and compulsive behaviors.

What all of these conditions have in common is a difficulty managing and regulating painful emotions. DBT assumes that people who are struggling with these conditions don't choose them. The assumption is that people either don't know what to do (a skills deficit) or forget what they know in an overwhelming moment. This analogy might help: It's one thing to not know *how* to swim (skills deficit) and then learn how to swim (skills acquisition); however, you might be a good swimmer, and yet it is difficult to use the skill if you are thrown into the Atlantic Ocean in the middle of a raging storm.

How Does DBT Work?

DBT helps people focus on accepting and validating the challenges that bring them into therapy. At the same time, it encourages people to change their behaviors by using new skills to deal with life's problems, focusing on what you can do *in the here and now* to be more effective in your life. DBT is typically offered either as individual or group therapy, or both.

Individual therapy. In the early stages of therapy, you might go twice per week and start with a focus on self-destructive behaviors. That might be frustrating, since there is so much to talk about! However, talking about difficult things can actually increase emotional intensity, and if you don't know what to do with strong emotions, this can lead to dangerous behaviors. Typically, a person in DBT keeps track of their behaviors and the things they are working on by using a diary card, and the individual brings the diary card for review in each session.

Skills training groups. Here, others who are participating in DBT therapy join with others in a group to learn the actual skills, and research shows that it is the learning of new skills that seems to be the most important element of the treatment.[4] So if you can't find an individual DBT therapist but can find a group, join the group! Of course, if you are struggling with suicidal and self-destructive behaviors, having an individual DBT therapist is ideal.

What Are the DBT Skills?

There are four skill sets that are taught in DBT, and these focus on the problems that bring people into DBT therapy.

Mindfulness. This is the practice of being fully present and aware, and doing so without being judgmental. The concept is simple, and yet it is easier said than done because the mind is easily distracted by thoughts that take us to the past or to fears about the future. However, like most skills, the more you practice, the easier it will be. Mindfulness is a key practice because many people who come to DBT spend a lot of time dwelling in the suffering of past hurts and traumas, or worrying about a future that has not yet happened.

But when we settle ourselves in the present, our perspective becomes clearer, and we can plan more effectively. Mindfulness helps manage strong emotions, tolerate difficult moments more effectively, and improve and enhance relationships.

Try It: A short, simple mindful grounding exercise is to just notice and name each of your five senses. Name one thing you can hear, one you can taste, one you can smell, one physical sensation, and one interesting new visual element in the environment around you.

Distress tolerance. There are many times when we can't solve problems in the moment, or at least, the solutions we have may not be the healthiest in the long run. The distress tolerance skills teach you to manage stressful moments more effectively, while preserving your self-respect. These might include things like taking one small step to make the moment better, self-care, making a list pros and cons of engaging in behaviors, doing some relaxation practices, or volunteering. It also involves recognizing that although behaviors like substance use can help you tolerate distress in the immediate moment, they often causes more problems in the long run.

Try It: Building on the five senses exercise above, try doing something to stimulate yourself in a positive way with your five senses. For example, try eating a delicious snack, enjoying the comforting sensations of a warm shower or applying smooth lotion, smelling a favorite candle or essential oil, listening to soothing music or nature sounds, or looking at beautiful artwork or other images.

Interpersonal effectiveness. These skills help you get more of what you want out of relationships without alienating people. They can help you repair relationships, set better boundaries, and take perspective, especially if someone else's behavior is confusing. The most important of the skills is self-validation, where you recognize that your experience, including suffering, makes sense and is valid. Validation is a skill that we therapists use a lot and work toward having our patients be able to do for themselves.

Emotion regulation. This skill set teaches all about what emotions are, how they can help us, and how to manage them. You learn to reduce your vulnerability to strong emotions and how to increase positive emotions. It breaks down emotions into their component parts, meaning the associated thoughts, body sensations, and urges, so that you have a better ability to deal with them. For example, saying that you are sad that you weren't invited to a party is clearer than saying that you are overwhelmed by social situations.

A popular emotion regulation skill is known as *opposite action.* Here's an example: Say you are feeling sad and your urge is to isolate and stay in bed in your dorm in your pajamas. This behavior does not generally make anyone feel happy, even if temporarily it feels good to avoid everything. In fact, in the long term, you are likely to become more depressed. Using *opposite action* would be to do something opposite (or different) to your action urge and so the behavior would be to get up, take a shower, and call a friend. Yes, it can feel exhausting if you're down, but staying in bed and isolating will almost certainly not make you feel better.

DBT can be helpful even without a specific diagnosis.

I had never heard of DBT, but I went to a DBT group on campus and honestly felt like everyone should learn it. It's like taking a life 101 course, helpful with emotions, with relationships, with boundaries. I use the skills almost every day at work and in my regular life, even years after that group sophomore year.
                    —Grace, recent graduate now working in health care

What Is Acceptance and Commitment Therapy?

Mindfulness is a key element of many new therapies, including acceptance and commitment therapy (ACT), developed by Steve Hayes in the 1990s. ACT is also about action and learning how not to "believe everything you think." A key element to the approach is *acceptance*—we accept that we are anxious about the semiformal, rather than wasting energy trying to fight it or bail. The next step is to channel the energy saved in fighting reality to help you focus, and even recognizing that if you are anxious, that you are also excited. Both can be true.

Another aspect of ACT is what's called "cognitive defusion," where you learn to see your negative thoughts as just thoughts. One example is to write them down on paper and then hold the paper at a distance, or repeat them over and over until they hold less power over you.

ACT also emphasizes your lifelong goals and values are beyond the upcoming weekend or midterms. It involves reminding yourself that each day you're moving toward both immediate goals like school and your lifelong goals. Lastly, *committed action* is about *acting your way into a new way of thinking, not just trying to think your way into a new way of acting.* It's feeling the fear and doing it anyway. It's showing up at the party if you're nervous, giving the class presentation even if you don't want to, and showing up to the club even when you don't know anyone.

A lot of students find ACT to work well and find the exercises and homework to be interesting, even fun, and the new skills to be applicable in many aspects of life. For more, check out books like *Get out of Your Mind and Into Your Life* by Steven Hayes.

What Is Positive Psychology?

Positive psychology starts with the premise that there is more right in your life than is wrong in your life, and that you can effectively leverage strengths to help yourself overcome challenges. Not all therapies work for everyone. In part, it depends on what you need. Some skeptics dismiss positive psychology as "toxic positivity," but when it's done right, it can be incredibly empowering. Oftentimes evidence-based practices like the ones we just reviewed include elements of positive psychology, with a focus on your existing strengths. One way that we as therapists integrate this is to get our patients to reflect on what got them through hard times in the past, consider what positive attributes they have, and encourage them to reflect on the likeable qualities others appreciate about them. The approach is not for everyone, and certainly if you are depressed, anxious, or have issues around self-esteem, positive psychology can feel challenging.

Here are a few exercises:

1. Positive psychology also involves practices like making a list of what is going well in your life, as well as a list of struggles. By writing the positives, you are overcoming what is known as a "negativity bias." Almost all of us will have negative thoughts at some point, and this is true particularly when we feel depressed or anxious. When you're feeling this way, try making a list of some pleasurable events and helpful encounters or people that you have experienced in the last two days.
2. Another concrete action you can take is to understand your strengths. Take the Penn Positive Psychology Strengths Inventory (https:// positivepsychology.com/via-survey/) and see what you come up with. Reviewing your strengths can really impact your mood and outlook.

My favorite class I took so far was an elective in positive psychology. It was called the science of happiness or something and was honestly life changing. I can't recommend it enough . . . we even tried to start a positive psychology club on campus.

—Ezra, senior at a medium-sized city university

What Are Mind-Body Approaches to Mental Health?

Mind-body approaches work on the premise that a healthy body leads to a healthy mind and that a healthy mind leads to a healthy body. They focus less on talking as therapy and more on doing. They might include breath regulation practices, yoga, martial arts, and other forms of exercise.

Biofeedback and Neurofeedback

Biofeedback is the use of noninvasive monitoring equipment and instruments to measure your body's involuntary functions, including your heart rate, blood pressure, breathing rate, and muscle tension. By using the data from the equipment, you recognize that there are biological clues that you might not be aware of. For instance, say that you are talking about a former romantic partner, and your heart rate goes up and your muscles become tense. By making these things conscious, your therapist can suggest techniques to relax, and you can take previously unconscious information and make voluntary and intentional changes.

A related technique is neurofeedback, which is used to help teach control of brain functions by identifying brain waves that can indicate a state of attention or inattention. Over time, when you are losing attention, you learn to recognize that you are doing so because your brain waves that focus on attention are less active. This can be useful for conditions like attention-deficit/hyperactivity disorder (ADHD).

> My parents sent me to do biofeedback when I was in middle school, and it helped me a ton with anxiety and insomnia I had been having back then. I still use the relaxation skills I learned back then in college now when the stress is too much.
> —Gabe, economics major at a large southern public university

Mind-Body Exercises

Breathwork
7/11 Breathing. When you regulate your breath, you regulate your attention, impulses, and emotions. Try slowing it down to about five or six a minute, to really activate calm and clarity. There are many variations, but one is 7/11 breathing. Breathe in through your nose to the count of 7 and then out through pursed lips to the count of 11. Try this for five breath cycles. What changes did you notice?

Posture Changes

Just as your mood changes, so does your posture. For instance, maybe you look down and hunch over when you are sad or jumping for joy when you are happy. Changing your body posture can change your mood.

Try this: Place your hands behind your head and lean back. This stretches and relaxes the vagus nerve—important in the fight/flight response, as well as automatically deepening and slowing the breath. If you notice it helping, try it every few questions during a test!

Power Poses

According to Harvard researcher Amy Cuddy,[5] changing your posture to a confident "power pose" can help boost confidence, wash out stress-related cortisol, and activate hormones like testosterone, which can improve self-confidence. One form of power pose is to stand or sit consciously in an open posture with your shoulders back, eyes looking forward (not at the ground), and palms facing slightly outward. Try it.

What Is Eye Movement Desensitization and Reprocessing?

Eye movement desensitization and reprocessing (EMDR) is a therapy initially developed for the treatment of trauma, but it is now in use for a number of other mental health issues. It is based on a theory that shows that "bilateral stimulation," meaning stimulation of both sides of your brain, can help people process traumatic events in a way that traumatic memories no longer hold power over the person.

> I went to regular therapy about the trauma of a harassment situation that had happened to me back in high school with my field hockey coach, and it was really helpful to understand myself and my reactions. The therapist also suggested I do EMDR, and I tried it a few times and found it helpful for managing the trauma as well. It was just a few sessions while I continue to work with my regular therapist.
>
> **—Kai, first-year student at small liberal arts college**

What Are Family Therapy and Couples Therapy?

These treatment modalities can be useful if you have unresolved family issues, and they can often be scheduled when you are home for the summer between academic years. Family therapy is used to focus on better ways of communicating and expressing needs and setting boundaries more effectively. It is also useful for setting effective limits and typically involves at a minimum two members of the family.

Couples therapy might also be helpful, even if it only entails one or two sessions with a romantic partner. Similar to family therapy, it can help educate loved ones on how to be supportive, how the mental health issues impact you or your loved one, and how to ask for what you need and set clear boundaries.

> My boyfriend who has BPD [borderline personality disorder] invited me into one session with his therapist, and I learned a lot about how I could better support him, but also how I could take better care of myself. Like, a bit more about when I could say no if he needed emotional support which made my life easier, feeling like I wasn't always responsible for him and his emotions, and it wasn't my fault if he self-harmed or went back to cocaine.
>
> —Lauren, junior at a small public college

There's also no rule against other people coming to your therapy a few times, or more. You might want to invite your parents, partner, siblings, or even college friends to some appointments to help sort things out.

> I 100% dreaded the family meetings that I knew were coming at the end of my time in the hospital program. They were not exactly fun. But I will say I'm really glad that I did those family sessions because even though my parents and I aren't on the exact same page, they understand how to support me so much better than they did before I went into the hospital, and it's really taken care of one the biggest stresses I had before my depression got so bad.
>
> —Jasmine, recent graduate

What Is Internal Family Systems?

Internal Family Systems (IFS) is a form of psychodynamic therapy that's been growing in popularity. Developed by Richard Schwartz, it is built on the idea that we all say things like "Part of me wants to take the semester off, and part of me wants to stick it out," and then working with those different parts, by putting them into conversation with each other while the therapist focuses on the typical patterns you seem to get stuck in.

Try It: Say you want to stay in bed. Can you validate and recognize the parts of yourself that want to stay in bed, the parts of you that want to hang out with friends, and the parts that want to get out and go to class? Listen deeply to the parts that want to go to class, the parts that want to see friends, and the parts of you that don't want to leave your bed. See if you can recognize the motivations of each part from a place of nonjudgment and compassion.

What Is Spiritual Counseling?

In many respects, spiritual and religious counseling is the original therapy. Before psychotherapy and psychoanalysis were developed, people would approach a priest, guru, astrologer, or spiritual advisor to get advice, develop a deeper self-understanding, and get relief from suffering. For some of us, our anxieties or feelings of depression come from the big existential questions: Who am I? Why am I here? What is my purpose in this world? And spiritual counseling can, at times, provide more satisfying answers and grounding practices to what feels beyond our control or understanding.

Many students and their families may seek out spiritual counseling that feels more resonant with their faith, and if faith is important, we strongly encourage you to do so as well. Having someone who understands how you make sense of the world can be helpful as it relates to your spiritual beliefs. The campus chaplains are often trained in some spiritual counseling, or you can reach out to clergy from back home if you've had a strong relationship with them over time as well.

> I stayed in touch with my pastor from back home, which was incredibly helpful in the first year of college to feel that connection, especially on a pretty secular campus. But when things got hard junior year, he helped me get connected with more traditional counseling up here which I didn't realize how much I needed until I started.
>
> —Jessica, junior at a large public university

What Are Arts and Expressive Therapies?

Arts and expressive therapies are gaining more traction and recognition in psychotherapy. Research shows that it is possible to dance, draw, paint, and sculpt your way to feeling better emotionally. It isn't as simple as opening your sketchbook and drawing. Your therapist has been trained to offer specific exercises and focus on how your creative expression can help you process your emotions or come to a greater sense of self-understanding.

What Is Group Therapy?

Different colleges focus on therapist-led groups, rather than offering individual therapy. Groups are recommended because you can often learn a lot from other people who have "been there, done that" and work with other group members who share ideas on shared experiences. Peer support can also help hold you accountable to your commitments. Helping others also boosts self-esteem and recovery, and in so doing, you can see how far you've come and how much you have to offer.

At school or locally, there may be affinity support groups for certain students with certain mental health issues or marginalized identities. Groups also might be very structured for a set period of time, say five weeks, or might be more open ended.

In Conclusion

We hope this is a good introduction to some of the most popular and researched options that are out there, and there are, of course, plenty more. We encourage you to explore more, especially if what you're doing now is not working for you. And the reality is that you might not find a perfect fit in terms of therapy. Don't be afraid to bring this up—a good therapist won't be defensive and will be able to shift gears to help you get what you do need, or be able to refer you to someone else who can be more supportive.

Chapter 5
Medication

What's the Role of Medication in Mental Health?

Not everyone needs psychiatric medication as a way to help their mental health, and you might have some worry or skepticism yourself. We do, too. No medication, just like no psychotherapy, is a magic bullet. Although they can be extremely helpful in certain psychiatric conditions, medications are not for everyone. And when they do work, they tend to work best in conjunction with talk therapy. Also, even if you might benefit from an antidepressant for low-grade depression, many research studies show that alternatives to medication are just as effective. For instance, a meta-study that reviewed many other studies on the effects of a physical exercise intervention on depressive and anxious moods in college students[1] showed that 30 minutes of exercise a day was effective in reducing depression and anxiety. In another study comparing exercise to antidepressants,[2] the authors concluded that exercise is 1.5 times more effective at reducing mild-to-moderate symptoms of depression, psychological stress, and anxiety than medication *or* cognitive behavioral therapy.

Given that not all mental health conditions need medication and, furthermore, that there are circumstances when getting a prescription might be difficult, in addition to the expense and some undesirable side effects, how do you decide when medication is essential versus when there are other options to treat your mental health issues?

What Factors Should I Consider?

These are general guidelines, and ideally you are discussing these with a prescriber, mental health specialist, your family doctor, your parents, and/or your school counseling center.

1. **Side effects.** All medications can have side effects, and, depending on the type of medication, you may experience none, mild, moderate, or severe side effects. If the medication is causing significant side effects and does not appear to be helping the underlying mental health condition, it may not be worth taking. If the medication is helping, then speak to your prescriber to see if there can be a way to address the side effects. Also, some medications can lead to conditions such as obesity or diabetes, and these are important to consider if you have these conditions in your family, or if you are at risk for them. Other side effects may emerge when taken with other medications, or when taken with recreational substances, so be sure to consider with your prescriber before you take anything else with your medication.

2. **Delay in onset.** It can take weeks to know whether a psychiatric medication is working. If your current medication isn't working, then the next medication may take weeks to test out. For that reason, you may not want to experiment with trials during college. Ask yourself if you can deal with the level of distress in the moment, and if you can, can you wait for a school break to try a new medication? If medications are going to take four to six weeks to work and have side effects, you may be getting all of the negatives and none of the positives while you are trying to be a student. In other cases, is it worth it? And, of course, you can always chat with your advisor, dean, and/or professor to sort out how to best navigate any of the ways that this new medication might impact your academic performance.

3. **Effectiveness.** We see many students who have been taking medication for years. In some cases, they do not think that the medication is helping at all. If a student is feeling stable and is on multiple medications, it may be because the medication is actually helping. However, many doubt that they are helping and have the urge to simply stop. *Do not stop medication without speaking to your prescriber!* Stopping medications can be done safely and carefully with the help of a prescriber, who typically recommends that you reduce medications slowly and one at a time, rather than all medications at once. Your brain is used to being on medication so stopping them suddenly can cause serious complications. Remember

also that your brain and body are continuing to change all the time, even through the college years, and this may impact the efficacy of the medications as well.

4. **Medications are not a cure**. Psychiatric medications are not like antibiotics, which can cure an infection after a round of usage. Although psychiatric medications can treat many of the symptoms of mental illness, they do not cure mental illness, and many people have to take psychiatric medications on and off over a lifetime. In many situations, medications can be lifesavers. However, if you are not in immediate danger, take your time to decide and explore your options. And remember that for many conditions, our ancestors did not have psychiatric medications, and they used other methods to manage their mental health, which we describe in Chapter 6. Also note that sometimes taking the medication is not enough. You might benefit from the medication *and* engaging in self-care activities, seeking therapy, or other supportive measures.

5. **Brain plasticity**. Tina Bryson also reminds us that the brain is especially "plastic" at your age, meaning it is changeable. Your current experiences will shape your brain for the rest of your life. That's why even taking medication to get through a hard time in the college years can actually change the trajectory of mental illness, because the medication can allow you to access the therapy and other skills and strategies that will set you on a path toward thriving mental health for a lifetime. Then, perhaps it'll be easier to taper off of the medication and manage on your own. It's almost like a primer coat of paint, so the talk therapy can stick better, and then your brain can potentially set in a positive mold for the rest of your life. Sometimes this is called the "kindling effect," where the issues worsen unless treated early—catch the fire before it gets out of control. The medication lets the support work; it's not either/or.

With all this in mind, here is what the research shows for various conditions:

- **For depression**: Cognitive behavioral psychotherapy and interpersonal psychotherapy, together with antidepressant medications, have been shown to be helpful. However, some studies show that therapy alone can help, and as we reviewed, exercise might be better than medication for mild to moderate depression. Certainly, for people who have severe depression, or who are hearing voices or are suicidal, medication is strongly recommended.

- **For anxiety disorders**: Cognitive behavioral therapy together with antidepressant and antianxiety medications have all been shown to be helpful. Research shows that therapy is more effective than medication and that adding medication to therapy does not significantly improve outcomes. Again, interventions like exercise and other forms of therapy, such as exposure therapy, can be more useful than medication.
- **For alcohol and substance use disorders**: Cognitive behavioral therapy and environment-based therapies, as well as 12-step support programs, have been shown to be helpful. For some people in the early phases of withdrawal or treatment, medications that reduce cravings can be helpful. When these are used, a person does not typically have to be on them for the rest of their life.
- **For eating disorders**: Different forms of behavioral therapy and environmental interventions are the standard treatment. For people with severe eating disorders, such as medically significant anorexia, the addition of antipsychotic medication, which can help with delusional thinking and stimulate appetite, can be helpful. Typically, these medications are not long term.
- **For schizophrenia or bipolar disorder**: Most people with these conditions do require medication, and it could be dangerous not to use them. Research suggests that adding cognitive behavioral therapy to the treatment can improve functional outcomes.
- **For borderline personality disorder or self-injury**: There are no medications, and dialectical behavior therapy and other psychotherapies are the treatment of choice. Medications are useful when there are comorbidities, meaning other mental health disorders that can be treated by medication, as well in situations where a person is severely agitated and one or two days of a medication could be helpful to get through the crisis.

The Use of Medication on College Campuses

Although the majority of college students do not take psychiatric medications, there are many who do, and the numbers are rising. In a recent study[3] that reviewed the use of medication use on campuses from 2007 to 2019, there was an increase in use of nearly all types of psychiatric medications. Antidepressant medication use increased from 8.0% to 15.3%, antianxiety medication increased from 3.0% to 7.6%, stimulant medication increased from 2.1% to 6.3%, antipsychotic medication from 0.38% to 0.92%, and mood stabilizers from 0.8% to 2.0%. Many students are also taking more than one type of medication. In 2007, 28% of students on medications took more than one medication type, and this has risen to more than 40%. It's likely these numbers have only increased. The bottom line is that if you take psychiatric medications, you are not alone.

Can I Take Someone Else's Medication?

A recent survey sponsored by the National Institute of Health (2023)[4] found nearly 17% of college students reported using one or more types of prescription drugs that either they themselves had *not* been prescribed or were being used for nonmedical reasons. The survey also reported that college students have a higher likelihood of misusing prescription stimulants when compared to same age peers who are not in college. Many of these medications are obtained from other students who do have a legitimate prescription. This also means that the students who have a legitimate prescription are not using them as directed, or that if they are supposed to be taking them daily, but are giving some of them to other students, that the student will run out of the medication ahead of time.

Looking more closely at the numbers, a researcher[5] found the following:

- **Frequency of misuse**: 6.8% of students reported misusing pain medications, 7.8% reported misusing sedatives, and 14.5% reported misusing stimulants.
- **Access to prescription drugs**: 11.4% of students said it was easy to obtain pain medication for recreational use; 15.2% of students said that it was easy to get sedatives; and 26.4% of students said it was easy to get stimulant medications. The majority of students who misuse prescription drugs say that they typically get the drugs from other students— 44.0% for pain medications, 54.6% for sedatives, and 76.9% for stimulants.
- **Reasons for use**: The most common reasons that students said that they misused pain medications were to get high (46.0%) and to relieve pain (40.8%); sedatives were misused to relieve anxiety (50.8%) or as sleep aids (47.3%); and stimulants were to study or improve grades (76.1%). It is important to know that there is no evidence that students who do not need stimulants and yet misuse them in order to get better grades do *not* get better grades and in many instances have episodes of heart palpitations and anxiety as a side effect.

- **Prescribed medication behaviors**: Only 8.6% of students said that they kept their prescription drugs in a safe, locked space; the majority said that they kept their medications in an unlocked medicine cabinet or desk or dresser drawer. This point is very important as we have heard that medications that have not been properly stored have been ingested or stolen by other students.

Is Medication a Cure-All?

Most students who struggle at school and college, or even seek counseling, don't necessarily have a formal psychiatric condition. Still, many have a history of depression, anxiety, and other diagnoses before they even go. In just 2022, more than three-quarters of college students experienced significant psychological distress, and 35% of students were diagnosed with anxiety and 27% had depression.

This means that many students will be taking medication, and there are a few important aspects to consider. This medication section is divided into a few sections. The first is practical and general considerations, and the second covers specific classes of medication and their role in mental health treatment. The following sections review these important considerations.

Transition From Home to College

Many of the students we work with can't wait to leave home. It's a key, and developmentally appropriate, step to a life of increased autonomy. And yet with increased autonomy comes increased responsibility, and one such responsibility is managing medication. Often, high school seniors still have parents deciding on their medications, as well as prepacking their medication cassettes and reminding them to take the pills.

Ideally, any child or young adolescent should know the medications they are taking, but for those heading off to college, certainly by their senior year of high school a student should be clear as to what their medications are, the doses they take, for what symptoms or diagnoses, at what time of day, potential side effects, how to manage refills, what the local pharmacy hours are, what the co-pay for medication is, and so on.

WORKSHEET

- My medications and doses are:

_____

_____

_____

_____

- I take them at the following times:

_____

_____

_____

_____

- For the following diagnosis/diagnoses:

_____

_____

_____

_____

- Side effects to watch out for:

_____

_____

_____

_____

- Past trials of medications that have not worked for me are:

_____

_____

_____

_____

- I can get multiple refills for the following medications:

_____

_____

_____

_____

- I need a monthly prescription for the following medications:

_____

_____

_____

_____

- My prescriber is, and their phone number is:

_____

_____

_____

_____

- My local pharmacy is:

_____

_____

_____

_____

- Their hours of operations are:

_____

_____

_____

_____

- The co-pay for my medication is:

_____

_____

_____

_____

If for the first few months of high school the student struggles with managing their medications, parents can walk through the steps necessary and increasingly hand the responsibility to their adolescents. By the time they get to college, both parent and college student should feel confident that they can manage the logistics of their medications.

Access to a Prescriber

There are many elements to take into account when considering a prescriber. For many students, their home prescriber is comfortable continuing to prescribe the medication, especially if the student is on stable and effective doses of medication, with no or few side effects. Students either see their prescribing clinician when they come home during breaks or check in by phone or video call. However, some prescribing clinicians are prevented by their licensing board or institutions from prescribing or seeing patients across state lines. Other medications are controlled and can't be prescribed in longer doses than a month. They may be happy to see the student over break but ask them to find a prescriber in the state where they are going to school. Check as soon as you decide on a school so that you can make a decision. This is for two reasons: The first is that because there is such a high demand for psychiatrists and other prescribers, there may be a long waiting list near your school. The second is that once a prescriber has been identified, your prescriber can share clinical information with the new person.

CHECKLIST

☐ Can my prescriber work with me even when I am out of state? If yes, then you are all set. If no, then:

☐ As early as I know that I will need a new prescriber, I need to start calling around. Often, college counseling centers have a prescriber on staff, and you will need to see if the college you are going to does have one. Does my college have a prescriber on staff? If yes, you are all set. If no, then:

☐ You can make your own calls to local area psychiatrists or ask the counseling center if they have a list of local prescribers. You will also need to check to see if the prescribing clinician takes your insurance or the college insurance.

☐ If, despite all your efforts, you simply cannot find anyone, and your medications are critical, you may want to prioritize colleges that are in or close to larger metropolitan areas where there will be greater access to prescribers, or you may need to come home more frequently in order to be seen by your local prescriber.

Access to a Pharmacy

You now know all about your medications and have ensured that either your current prescriber or a local psychiatrist is available to continue to prescribe. You now need to figure out where you will physically receive the medication.

Some national chains can transfer your information from a home pharmacy to one near school. If you are in a small town without a chain, you may need to switch to a local pharmacy. This typically means calling the pharmacy and giving them your insurance information and a credit card for co-pays. Co-pays are the amount of money you will need to pay beyond what your insurance covers. This can range from a few dollars to up to a hundred dollars. You will need to find that out. We have seen students learn that their co-pay was beyond what they had in their account and then have to scramble to either (1) find some way to pay for the medication, or (2) consider switching to a cheaper medication. You might want to check if the pharmacy is a 24-hour pharmacy.

The easiest option is finding out if your pharmacy will deliver to your college or even to your dorm. If you are comfortable with this, just be sure you've got your address correct!

Many students don't want others to know or find out that they are taking psychiatric medication. In one study of nearly 4,000 students, 17.6% of the students had taken psychiatric medication in the last year. Of these students, 22% received their medications on campus, 61.7% received their medications off campus, and 6.4% received them both on and off campus. Unfortunately, nearly 10% of students took medications without a prescription, and we strongly recommend against this. The bottom line is that many students prefer to pick up the medication themselves and do so at the off-campus pharmacy.

CHECKLIST

- ☐ Is there a local pharmacy where I can pick up my medications?
- ☐ Establish an account with your insurance information and a credit card for co-pays.
- ☐ What is the co-pay for my medication?
- ☐ What are their hours of operation, or are they a 24-hour pharmacy?
- ☐ Alternatively, does my college have an option to receive the medication in the health center? Or am I comfortable having the medication delivered at my dorm?

Storing the Medication

You now know all about your medication, who is going to be prescribing the medication, and where you will pick it up or how it will be delivered. How do you store the medication? Here are things to consider:

First, you should let your college health center know that you are taking medication. This is so that they can take this into account, if you have any problems such as side effects, withdrawal effects, losing your medication, and so on. Some colleges recommend letting the dorm resident advisors (RAs) know.

Next is storage. Many dorm rooms are easily accessible, and you or your roommate might leave your door open or unlocked. Unfortunately, some medications can be abused, typically those in the stimulant and tranquilizer class, and you'll need to be careful to ensure they aren't taken by others. Some colleges provide safe storage in the dorms, but you might want your own storage device. Some students hide their medication, but if you hide them too well, you might forget where you have hidden them or forget to take them altogether. If you are someone who tends to forget, establishing effective daily routines and alarms are essential. Certainly, if your college is close to home, you may choose to leave the bulk of your medication at home and pick up what you need every week or every two weeks.

CHECKLIST

- ☐ Have I let the college know that I take medication if any issue regarding the medication arises?
- ☐ Does my college or dorm have a safe storage option for medications?
- ☐ Do I have a medication storage device that is safe and can easily be hidden from view?

☐ If I tend to be someone who forgets to take their medications, what is my plan for developing habits that will ensure that I reliably take my medication?

☐ Do I know what to do if I forget a dose or lose my meds? Where should I keep my medication?

You need to know that certain environmental factors can damage your medications; in particular light, heat, and moisture. In college, you need to take the extra precaution of storing them in a place where they are not visible to others, so that they will not be tempting to others. This is particularly true if you share a room with others. Remember that a lot of drug experimentation takes place on campuses, and your roommates might want to experiment with your prescription medication.

Store your medications in a cool, dry place. If you have a lock box, that would be ideal. Put it in a place that is not clearly visible. If you are used to storing your medication above the sink in your bathroom cabinet, or you have a cabinet above your sink, or in your bathroom if you live off campus, remember that heat and moisture from your shower or bath can damage the medication.

Another important point is to always keep your medication in its original container. Here is the experience of a student who did not do this:

I didn't want my roommates to know that I was on stimulants, so I took out my Ritalin and put it in an antihistamine bottle because I also get congested. Anyway, one of my roommates told me that there was something wrong with him. He said that he had been up all night for the past three nights, that he could not sleep, and that he had been making up sonnets. He was worried that he was having a nervous breakdown. We took him to the on-campus clinic, and they asked him if he was taking any drugs or medication. He said: "No, the only thing I've taken is my roommate's decongestant because I think I have allergies." I was horrified and I told the nurse and my roommate about my meds and putting them in a different bottle. Now it's kinda funny, but it could have been really bad!

—Yaron, sophomore at a medium-sized city university

Action Items

- Do I have a place to safely store my medication?
- Is it cool and dry?
- Is it visible to anyone entering my room?
- Is my medication in its original container?

Old Medication

It is important not to take medication that has expired or that is damaged. Time can degrade medication and make it lose its potency. This can be particularly important for medications such as birth control that, if damaged or expired, can become almost completely ineffective.

- Don't take medication that has changed color or texture, or that sticks together.
- If you have expired or damaged medications, take them to your local pharmacy. Not all pharmacies have a disposal program, but they might tell you how to dispose of them safely.
- Don't flush old medications down the toilet or sink, as you'll possibly be introducing medication into the water supply chain.

Traveling With Medicine

By car: Do not keep medicine in the glove compartment of your car. Medicine can get too hot or humid in there and change its efficacy and it may be tempting for someone else to take it if they open the compartment.

By plane: Although you can travel with most medication, make sure that they are kept in the original bottles. There are some medications that are liquid or injectable, and as long as they are properly labeled and you have a prescription from your doctor, you will be allowed to pass through security with them. For instance, some people with diabetes might need syringes, needles, and lancets to test their blood sugar and inject insulin. Some antibiotics are in liquid form. Some psychiatric medications are formulated in liquid form because some people have a hard time swallowing pills.

Ensuring Timely Delivery of Refills

You know what your medications are, who prescribes them, where to get them, and how to keep them. The last piece is getting the refills on time. Many psychiatric medications can be prescribed for a month with five refills. This means that as long as you are stable on your medication, there might not be a need to check in with your psychiatrist every month. If you are stable on your medication, it is reasonable to see your prescriber once every three months. However, some medications, known as controlled substances, medications that are considered by the Drug Enforcement Administration

(DEA) as having "a high potential for abuse which may lead to severe psychological or physical dependence," must be obtained every month, or at most every other month. You will need to determine this with your insurance company and your prescriber. It is critical that you stay on top of this, because not only will you need to pick up a prescription more often than your other medications, but if there are shortages, there may be even more challenges.

The bottom line is that you need to know if your medication requires monthly prescription or has automatic refills that do not need to be requested monthly. The other important factor is to see how many pills you have left for the month, and if you are running low, to see how many refills you have left.

CHECKLIST

- ☐ Does my medication need to be prescribed every month without refills?
- ☐ Does my medication allow for up to five refills (about a semester) without having to call my prescriber?
- ☐ How many pills do I have left for the month? When I have fewer than 10 pills, check the refill number, which is typically printed on the medication bottle.
- ☐ If my medication allows for refills, how many refills do I have left?
- ☐ If I have zero or one refill, I should call my prescriber?

Some Other Ideas

We have now covered all the major situations that can arise, but here are a few other tips. If you tend to forget taking your medications in the morning, some students have told us that they keep their medications in their toiletry or shower kit so that they see it when they go to brush their teeth in the morning. Smartphone alarms can be helpful for reminders, especially if the medications are taken at a specific time of day. Use a unique tone or song to distinguish it from your morning alarm.

Never Experiment With Prescription Drugs

If you have never taken psychiatric medication, but you are struggling with mental health concerns and you are considering if they might be helpful, *do not* experiment with medications that others are taking "just to see." At a fundamental level, the medication might not be helpful, but it could be worse; you might develop severe side effects, including significant weight gain, sedation, confusion, anxiety, and other problems. If you are considering medication, this is something you will need to speak to a prescriber about. If you don't have a prescriber, many counseling centers have prescribers they can recommend.

Once you meet with a prescriber, be sure to tell them anything else you take, from vitamins and supplements, alcohol and recreational drugs, to prescription drugs for other conditions as these can interfere or interact with psychiatric medications.

If you cannot find a psychiatrist, some primary care physicians are willing to prescribe. Even if you cannot find an MD, there are other non-MD clinicians who can prescribe psychiatric medication. In some parts of the country, there are very few psychiatrists. Psychiatric advanced practice nurses (APRNs) can prescribe as well, and in some states, physician assistants, under supervision, can also prescribe. There are a few states where the scarcity of psychiatrists is so significant that they allow for senior psychologists to prescribe, and these clinicians are known as prescribing or medical psychologists. You may want to check if this is an option if you have no other resources.

Next, we'll review the general classes of medications.

What Are the Specific Medication Classes?

The most commonly used prescription psychiatric medications on campuses are antidepressants, antianxiety medications, mood stabilizers, antipsychotics, and psychostimulants. This list is by no means exhaustive, nor do we endorse or recommend any of the medications listed. The specific medications listed are the ones most commonly taken by students. Of course, any medication decision should be made with your prescriber.

Important to know: Although medications are typically used for a specific condition, in many circumstances, psychiatrists will prescribe medications typically used for one category, for symptoms of another category. For instance, antidepressants might be used for anxiety, antipsychotics might be used to stabilize someone's mood, and so on.

Antianxiety Medications

Antianxiety medications are also known as anxiolytics. As their name implies, they are used to reduce the level of anxiety that you are experiencing. A significant problem with many of the medications in this class of drugs is that they can be powerfully habit-forming and can lead to dependence to the point of becoming a substance use disorder. For this reason, they're often only prescribed for a short period of time, even though we have seen many students who take them on a daily basis, for many months or even years.

The following are the different classes within this group:

Benzodiazepine: These medications work by increasing a chemical in the brain known as gamma-aminobutyric acid (GABA). The higher the level of GABA, the lower the level of brain activity, and this can help you feel calm and can make you sleepy. You can see how this type of drug could be very addictive. Some examples of the most commonly prescribed anxiolytics include alprazolam (such as Xanax), clonazepam (such as Klonopin), and lorazepam (such as Ativan).

Buspirone: This medication has been used for many years to treat chronic anxiety and panic attacks. It does not work immediately, and you will have to take it for a few weeks before you see full relief of symptoms. For this reason, many students don't want to take it, wanting immediate relief. However, because it is not habit-forming, it is a good option, especially if you are prone to addiction.

Beta-blockers: These drugs are commonly used as they can help reduce blood pressure. In psychiatry, they are prescribed to reduce the physical symptoms of anxiety and panic. They help for performance anxiety. Specifically, they reduce an elevated heart rate, sweating, and trembling. They are not addictive; however, because they can reduce blood pressure, sometimes to a dangerous level, blood pressure may need to be monitored. For some people, this class of medications can make them more depressed, which is obviously an unwanted side effect.

Antidepressants

Antidepressants, as their name implies, are used to treat depression; however, they are often used to treat other conditions. There are many different types of antidepressants, which is useful to know because if one antidepressant does not work, a different one might work. The most common classes of antidepressants are as follows:

Selective serotonin reuptake inhibitors (SSRIs): The theory behind these medications is that they steadily increase the amount of serotonin in your brain and that this increase helps to regulate the function of the nerves in your brain. Medications in this class include fluoxetine (such as Prozac), sertraline (such as Zoloft), and paroxetine (such as Paxil).

Selective norepinephrine reuptake inhibitors (SNRIs): These work by increasing the amount of norepinephrine in your brain. Norepinephrine increases your level of alertness, arousal, and attention. Medications in this class include venlafaxine (also known as Effexor) and duloxetine (also known as Cymbalta).

Bupropion: This medication is in a class of its own and seems to work by increasing both norepinephrine and dopamine in the brain. Beyond treating depression, it has been shown to be helpful in addiction.

If the antidepressants work, that is ideal; however, there are some important things you should know about antidepressants:

Sexual side effects: Antidepressants can cause significant sexual side effects. More than 50% of patients taking antidepressants complain of having no libido, or they say that they have pleasureless orgasms.

Quality of life: Ideally, by treating depression, a person's quality of life should improve; however, this is not necessarily true. A study[6] that analyzed nearly 9 million patients over an 11-year period concluded that people's quality of life does not improve over time.

Discontinuation syndrome: About 20% of people have a very difficult time stopping antidepressants because of the side effects. For some, the withdrawal effects are so bad that they cannot stop the medication even if the antidepressant is not working for depression.

The bottom line is that although antidepressants can help many people, they don't help everyone, and they can have some side effects that make depression worse.

Antipsychotics

As their name implies, antipsychotics are drugs used to treat psychotic conditions, which are disorders where a person cannot clearly tell the difference between reality and unreality. People with psychotic disorders hear voices that others cannot hear, see things that others cannot see, and experience enduring paranoia. Without this class of drugs, these conditions are so debilitating that many people would need around-the-clock psychiatric care. They are sometimes used to boost the effects of antidepressants, to treat mood disorders, and to reduce anxiety. There are two types of antipsychotics:

First-generation antipsychotics: These are also known as *typical antipsychotics* and are less commonly used today. They block the chemical pathways that cause hallucinations. Unfortunately, they can cause distressing side effects such as dry mouth and difficulty urinating, and when significant, they can cause significant problems in muscle coordination.

Second-generation antipsychotics: Also known as *atypical antipsychotics*, these are far more commonly used today in the treatment of psychosis and that is because they are considered to have fewer side effects. Some examples are clozapine (Clozaril), olanzapine (Zyprexa), risperidone (Risperdal), and quetiapine (Seroquel). Because of how they work in the brain, they have fewer side effects than the first-generation drugs. Nevertheless, there are some that you should know about. The following side effects are particularly concerning to the college student:

1. They can cause an increase in cholesterol and blood sugar; therefore, people with a predisposition to high cholesterol and diabetes should be particularly cautious and have regular blood tests.
2. They can cause dizziness and sedation, which can make it difficult to study.
3. They can cause weight gain.

Mood Stabilizers

As their name implies, mood stabilizers are medications that can reduce big mood swings, such as those that occur in the treatment of bipolar disorder (see Chapter 11). Mood stabilizers reduce the number and the intensity of mood swings. They can take up to several weeks to reach their full effect, and because of this, psychiatrists will often use antipsychotic and antianxiety medications in the early stages of acute bipolar disorder.

As with the other medications, there are different types of mood stabilizers in this class:

Lithium: This is the oldest and most studied of the mood stabilizers. To date, lithium is the gold standard for treating bipolar disorder. Like other medications, lithium has side effects. At higher doses, these include increased thirst and urination, nausea, weight gain, and hand tremors. Less common side effects include tiredness, blurred vision, impaired memory, difficulty concentrating, dry skin, and acne. Finally, some people experience thyroid and kidney function problems and, because of this, thyroid and kidney function are monitored regularly.

Anticonvulsants: These drugs were initially developed to treat epilepsy, but they also happen to be effective as mood stabilizers. The more common ones are lamotrigine (Lamictal), valproate (Depakote), and carbamazepine (Tegretol). Because valproate and carbamazepine can have more side effects than lamotrigine, they are less commonly used, and if they are used, they also require regular blood tests.

Psychostimulants

Stimulants are medications which are commonly used to treat attention-deficit/hyperactivity disorder (ADHD) and attention-deficit disorder (ADD). They work by increasing the amount of dopamine available to certain parts of the brain, which in turn increases alertness, focus, attention, and energy. A common myth is they make people smarter. *They do not!* Research shows that they do not help at all if you don't have ADD or ADHD. However, because they give students more energy, they are often misused.

There are two forms of stimulants:

1. **Immediate-release (short-acting)**: The effects of these can last for up to four hours. Some students will take these if they need to focus for short periods of time and they can be more flexible in when they take them as they will not impact sleep as much. Many students tell us that the downside is that once the medication wears off, they can experience an emotional crash where they notice a drop in energy and focus, and an increase in hunger and irritability.

2. **Extended-release (intermediate-acting or long-acting)**: These are typically taken once in the morning each day, although some students will take a break on weekends, especially if they don't need to study. The benefit of taking a break is that when they are restarted, there is less of a habituation effect. They can last from six to eight hours to as much as 16 hours. Longer-acting stimulants have fewer "ups and downs" than the short acting ones do; however, you have to be careful in that if you take them too late in the day, it may be nearly impossible to fall asleep.

As mentioned, psychostimulants can be very habit-forming and become drugs of abuse. There are also other side effects such as that they can temporarily cause appetite suppression, which can lead to rebound weight gain, and this is because when the stimulant wears off it can lead to bingeing and overeating. Another serious side effect is that they can cause significant insomnia. Perhaps the most serious side effect is that they cause an increase in dopamine, and this increase can be so significant that it can cause psychosis. Another concern is that because they are helpful in focusing a person's attention, they can cause hyperfocus to the point that you may lose creativity.

Psychedelics and Other Medications

Psychedelics have received a lot of attention in recent years. Early research on drugs like psilocybin[7] and MDMA[8] has shown they can help for depression and posttraumatic stress disorder (PTSD) even when other medications have failed. Many people use these drugs recreationally; however, there is no evidence that self-medicating with them is beneficial. Ketamine has been approved by the Food and Drug Administration (FDA), but it is different from other medications listed previously. Because it can affect a student's blood pressure and heart rate, it is delivered in a supervised clinical setting, and not all college campuses have, or are close to, a ketamine clinic. For some people, ketamine has been a life changer, and so if you need to be on ketamine, you should consider the proximity to a ketamine clinic in your school decision. If you want to consider a psychedelic class medication for mental health purposes, this must always be done through a licensed professional providing pharmaceutical-grade medication. There is never any assurance that psychedelic drugs obtained on campuses are pharmaceutical grade, that they are what they claim to be, or that they haven't been mixed with other drugs. Beyond ketamine, others drugs in this class are currently in development and undergoing trials and could become available in the near future.

What If Your New Provider Wants to Change Your Medication?

Once you get to college, and especially if you are going to college out of state, you might need to change providers. If your medications are stable, your new provider will likely continue prescribing what you are already on. Make sure your new and former prescribers are in touch in order to pass on necessary medical and medication information.

For many students, the right combination of medication has come after many trials and side effects to get to the point of stability. Still, sometimes a new prescriber will want to change your medication, and this can happen for many reasons:

1. The psychiatrist does not concur with your current combination of medications.
2. There are newer medications, with better evidence, and with fewer side effects.
3. They won't prescribe medications that are considered habit-forming, or potentially abusable, for more than a week or so at a time.
4. In their assessment, you have a different condition than what your home psychiatrist diagnosed you with.

Here is where your voice is extremely important: It is key that you communicate with your new psychiatrist and explain how it is that you landed on the medications that you are taking. How do you do this?

1. Be prepared for the possibility that the new prescriber wants to change medication. Review the Cope Ahead skill of DBT (see Chapter 6 in Chapter 4).
2. Have as complete a history of your past medication trials as possible; what worked, what didn't, what side effects you developed, and why they were prescribed.
3. Have your home prescriber's contact information ready, including the office phone number, fax number, and email, if that's the way they prefer to communicate. In this case, make sure that you have signed a release-of-information form in advance. This is a form that authorizes your providers to talk to each other.
4. If you feel stable on your medications and your new provider wants to change it up, be clear about how you feel. You can say something like: "I am worried about making changes right now. It took a long time to feel stable and get this combination right, and I am nervous that making changes just as I am starting college could make a difficult transition even harder.
5. If, for whatever reason, you cannot access your old records, you can reach out to your home pharmacy. Pharmacies should have records of medication going back years. They may not know why

you stopped or started them, but at least you will have the list. Your parents might also remember the effects and side effects of past medications.

6. Another reason that new prescribers may have concerns about your medication is that they have seen the impact of recreational drug and alcohol use on college students, and the facts show that nonprescribed drug use in college campuses is at all-time high,[9] and they may have concerns about the impact of alcohol and drugs interacting with your medication. This is particularly the case if you are already taking medications such as benzodiazepines or stimulants, which have abuse potential.

CHECKLIST

☐ If my home prescriber cannot prescribe out of state, do I have a new prescriber in college?

☐ Do I have a list of medications that I am currently taking?

☐ Do I have a list of my past medications, including what has worked and what has not worked?

☐ Do I have a list of the side effects or impact of past medication trials?

☐ Do I have the contact information for my current provider?

☐ Have I signed a release of information so that my home provider and new provider can talk?

☐ What is my Cope Ahead plan if the new prescriber wants to make medication changes?

☐ Do I have a list of side effects to watch for with my current medication, a plan for coping with them, and people who can help me keep an eye on them?

If your new prescriber strongly recommends that you change medication, there is often a good reason, and it is worth having the discussion. Hear them out and have an open mind to changes. For instance, on occasion we see students who were prescribed powerful antipsychotic medication that may have been helpful years ago but is no longer needed, and it may be causing side effects. If the new prescriber is familiar with your medication and can explain how they would monitor the changes, it may be worth considering. If you're not sure about the plan they are proposing, you can certainly let them know that you need to think about it, and you can likely call your home prescriber to get their opinion on the matter.

Remember, this is *your* brain and *your* mental health you are dealing with. *You* have the most to gain or lose. Don't be afraid to question changes to your plan, to advocate for yourself, to draw upon your support network for help, and if all else fails, to look for a different provider.

In Conclusion

If you take medication, you are definitely not alone. The number of college students who have taken psychiatric medications of all different classes has risen in the last decade; and many students are likely to be on more than one kind of psychiatric medication. Clearly, this means that the need for trained prescribers has increased and will likely continue to increase. The demands for such services will mean that you could find it very difficult to find timely help. Being prepared by reviewing the worksheets in this chapter and proactive by establishing connections and appointments many months ahead of landing on campus will save you a lot of frustration and is a true manisfetation of your commitment to your mental and overall health.

Chapter 6
Maintaining Your Gains and Self-Care

Why Does Self-Care Matter?

The notion of self-care is probably like an annoying broken record at this point, but it is for a reason. Self-care is important for everyone, but especially those struggling with mental health issues. When you take good care of your mind, body, and relationships, you build up a resilience (you could think of it like a psychological immune system) that can help keep your mental health issues at bay. The reality is, however, that it can be hard to maintain, especially as the semester goes on and work gets more intense, as well as social distractions and other commitments. We hope this chapter will offer you practical self-care tips along with routines. It can be particularly helpful to schedule your self-care time into your calendar or practice self-care with others to keep you motivated and help you remember. And if you do get out of the habit, please don't beat yourself up. Just try to get back into your healthy habits again. It happens!

How Do I Build a Support Network of People?

When you are struggling with mental health issues, it can feel *very* lonely and hard to know where to reach out for support. In fact, a recent study found that 51.5% of college students reported feeling lonely, so you are probably not as alone as you might think.[1] Yet it can be hard to remember this when our minds are crowded with negative distorted thoughts.

Dr. Tina Bryson reminds us that adversity plus support equals resilience, while adversity minus support equals fragility. We don't have to be alone with our pain, yet we know how much our mental illness tells us not to reach out.

In mental health, we talk about a "circle of care." Who is, or could be, in your circle of care? We've put together a list of potential options on your campus. We know that reaching out can be hard, but keep in mind that everyone on campus is basically there to support students in some way, so let them help you! Jot down a few ideas from this list of who might be most helpful for you. And we challenge you to reach out to even just one of them now. You've got this!

Social Connections
    Friends
    Roommates/housemates/hallmates
    Teammates
    Classmates
    Residential life staff
    Greek/social organizations
    Connections from extracurricular activities
    Co-volunteers at community service position
    Spiritual communities on campus
    Self-help communities on campus
    Coworkers at job
    Active minds and other mental health–oriented groups

Therapeutic Connections
    Campus counseling and therapy staff
    Campus medical staff
    Other students in campus support or recovery groups

Student Support Professionals
    Campus clergy
    Academic support professionals/tutors
    Career center staff
    Coaches

Staff at cultural and affinity centers
Campus ombudsperson
Title IX office
Financial aid office

Academic Supports
Advisors
Deans
Professors
Teaching assistants (TAs)

Off Campus
Support back home from family, friends, and others
Former teachers and coaches
Friends at other universities

What Is Real Self-Care?

Self-care, we want to be clear, is not self-indulgence with food, shopping, substances, and sex, although in moderation, those can be a welcome distraction. Nor is it self-denial, doing nothing but studying in the library and living like a monastic isolated scholar from the 15th century. True self-care is the steps you take to find balance when life is stressful, or before it might become so.

Following, we discuss biological, psychological, and social versions of self-care in terms of Maslow's Hierarchy of Needs as a frame. Maslow described all that a person needs to function, from basic physiological and safety needs, like food and shelter, to more complex needs, including love and belonging, self-esteem, and self-actualization. We'll break that down in a moment.

Physical Safety

Let's start with your body and physical safety, the foundation of mental health. Hopefully your tuition and room and board fees cover things like food, water, shelter, and sleep. Without those things, functioning at your best is going to be a real challenge. Many students are privileged enough to have these, but still, we've worked with many students with food and housing insecurity, who also struggle to afford warm jackets for New England winters. Under these conditions, focusing on mental health, to say nothing of academics, is difficult. Many schools have resources for students with financial hurdles to support these kinds of issues, so check in with financial aid, your dean or advisor, and the counseling or health center to see if they can point you in the right direction.

Sleep is included in this part of Maslow's hierarchy, too. Does your room feel safe, physically and emotionally, so you can truly rest there? Do you live in a situation where you can come back and take a nap if you need it? Sleep is a cornerstone to your emotional and physical well-being. Are you getting enough? Or, if you are not getting enough, is the quality of the amount of sleep you do get OK? It is better to get 6 hours of deep sleep than 10 hours of shallow, restless sleep, and that is because deep sleep offers specific physical and mental benefits, including the release of growth hormone, which helps to repair the microdamage that your muscle, bones, and other body tissues incurred during the day.

You should know that research has shown that you can't make up a "sleep deficit" by sleeping in all weekend. Ideally, try to go to bed and wake up at the same time every day. That puts less stress on your overall well-being. We know that's hard when you've got classes at all different times of day, or if you are up late with friends or studying, but try your best to prioritize it. Poor sleep is directly correlated with attention and memory issues, which will throw off your academics and make you feel depressed, anxious, and antisocial. Meditation and relaxation exercises can help, as might a few sleep aids such as melatonin, but check in with your prescriber before taking a sleep supplement or medication. Even 20 minutes of light exercise five days a week may be as good as medication for insomnia and has the added benefit of helping for some forms of depression, anxiety, and focus, too.

Eating three regular healthy meals a day is also going to keep your brain energized for managing your mental health and regulating your focus and emotions. Your class schedule may be tough in terms of regular meals and so, if you are going to be stuck studying in your room or in the library, you may want to keep some healthy snacks with you. Here's a tip: Many schools have a nutritionist on staff, and you might want to meet with them (especially if it's covered by your student health fees!).

And we will spare you the lecture on substances, but how you establish and stick with your own limits around substance use will also directly impact your physical (and mental) health and safety in the coming years. Ultimately this is your responsibility. Reflect for yourself on what your tolerance really is and what the impact of any potential overuse is. And remember, all the research says the longer you wait and less you use, the less likely you are to have a problem later in life.

The other things we tend to forget at college are some of the other medical basics. Especially if you're struggling with mental health, your medical health matters a lot! That's doubly true if you have chronic conditions like diabetes, allergies, or others that require regular medical check-ins. Get your annual physical from your pediatrician or doctor at home, or switch to local care or see someone at the health center on campus. Get your flu shot and any vaccinations—getting sick can exacerbate depression or anxiety, and it can lower your immune response, which can even reduce the amount you retain when learning! We've added a checklist below. Review it before you head to campus, and ideally, before you return each semester to ensure you're on top of things.

PHYSICAL HEALTH CHECKLIST

Do I have enough contact lenses, and is my eye prescription
up to date?   Yes ☐   No ☐

Do I need to make a dentist appointment?   Yes ☐   No ☐

Are there specialist appointments I need to plan for?   Yes ☐   No ☐

Do I have enough psychiatric *and* other regularly
taken medication?   Yes ☐   No ☐

Am I getting regular exercise, healthy food, and decent
sleep?   Yes ☐   No ☐

If I have severe allergies, or another potentially concerning
medical issue, do I have an alert bracelet and have I let the
health center know?   Yes ☐   No ☐

I have Type II diabetes, and basically when I got to college, I was still taking care of it, but not that well. I wasn't a big drinker before college, and even at college, but when I did drink, it threw my blood sugar off, which would impact my mood, anxiety, and focus. I actually ended up taking a semester off, sorting out my diabetes, and actually figuring out how to adapt my insulin better for weekends when I would be drinking a bit more, and went back to school in much better shape and better balanced than before.

—Scarlet, college graduate

In my time away from school, I started to notice how much the basics impacted my depression and anxiety. If I slept in, I actually got more depressed. If I slept not enough, I got anxious. I started setting alarms to wake up by ten—not super late for a college student, but my depression got better. I also noticed that when I ate three decent meals a day, I was less grouchy, or maybe I should say my parents and sister noticed that. I didn't want to hear it, but my therapist reminded me how important it was. And finally, I started getting even a little bit of exercise. I met with a trainer at my cheap gym, and got on a regular schedule of just doing the exercise bike for twenty minutes a few times a week, and noticed it also affected my mood. I'm just nervous about getting back to school and sticking to my routine, where I know it's going to be really hard.

—Mariana, taking a year off from school to work on mental health

We know these are hard habits to keep up, as Mariana shared. But that's also where friends and relationships (accountability buddies) can help. Best way to eat? Meet someone for lunch. Best way to exercise? Join a physical education class, yoga class, or meet a friend at the gym or for a run. Best way to sleep? Sometimes, in your roommate choosing process, you can indicate your sleep and scheduling needs and have them set you up with a roommate with similar needs (or they can help you move during the semester to live with someone else who does).

What Is Mindfulness?

Mindfulness practices have ancient roots stemming from religion and spirituality. In modern times, it has also been integrated into other activities, like sports and yoga, and is even used in therapies such as dialectical behavioral therapy (DBT) and acceptance and commitment therapy (ACT) (see Chapter 4). Why? It has extensive physical and mental health benefits, including better memory, greater ability to focus, better sleep, lower heart rate, reduced anxiety, a more effective immune system, a reduction in pain, and many others.

Although the instruction of mindfulness is quite simple, it can be hard to implement. The practice is to pay attention, to the here and now, with acceptance and without judgment. The reason that it is hard to implement is that we are constantly distracted by so many things, including incoming emails, texts, thoughts about what we need to do, memories of the past, and so on. When it comes to paying attention, research shows that mindfulness strengthens the circuits in the brain that are used for paying attention and focus. When you are focused on the present moment, rather than repeatedly reliving a painful past or fearing a future that has not yet arrived, you realize that you have a choice of where to put your attention, and for most people, any present moment is not the worst they have ever experienced. But focusing on the worst past moments or feared future moments taints the present moment with suffering.

When you practice mindfulness with acceptance and nonjudgment, you are not only accepting the present moment but also accepting yourself! Radical acceptance is not resignation, but learning to use your energy wisely, not fighting, running away, or just giving up, but instead embracing the perspective that in this moment, reality is as it is. The practice includes not judging yourself harshly and learning how not to believe critical inner voices.

Do you have a critical inner voice? What does it sound like and feel like to you?

_____

_____

_____

What Are Some Different Mindfulness Practices?

There are many types of mindfulness practices to choose from. For many people, the thought of mindfulness creates an image of a monk sitting in silent meditation. This is one type of meditation, but there are many others, including the following:

- Contemplative practices where you reflect on a question
- Guided practices where a teacher instructs you as you practice
- Moving practices where you focus on body movements like walking or yoga
- Generative practices where you focus on generating compassion for yourself and others
- In fact, anything you can do mindlessly, you can do mindfully! You can eat mindlessly while watching TV or focus on the taste of the food. You can talk to a friend with full attention, or you can do so while responding to your messages.

Now, because everyone is different, different mindfulness practices will work differently for different people. In the same way as there is not one way to exercise, there is not a singular approach to mindfulness. Yet in the same way that a part of exercise is to be healthier, part of mindfulness is to strengthen your ability to focus.

Mindfulness is a practice, and as with other practices, if you keep practicing, you will find that your ability to focus your attention, quiet your mind, be more effective in your relationships and reduce the intensity of emotions, will improve. There are near infinite mindfulness exercises, so here we will introduce some that you can try out:

1. **Sound grounding.** This practice can help you settle and help you focus, so it can be useful before an exam. Start by asking yourself, what's the farthest away sound that you can hear right now? Is it outside the room? In the yard? On the street? In the air?

   Next move to the nearest noises. Is there a fan? A door closing? Footsteps?

   Next see if you can hear noises your body is producing. Your stomach? Clothes rustling?

   Next, can you hear the sound of your breath?

   Now, switch your attention to sounds to your left and to your right. Above you and below you. In front and behind.

   This exercise is helpful for training to focus, and it is useful if your mind tends to wander, as well as to settle yourself or ground yourself.

2. **Feel your feet.** Our friend Jessica Morey at Rice University says that "if anxiety is in your head, focus on the farthest place: your feet," so take a moment to focus on your feet.

   A lot of people use this practice before public speaking, when trying to be more assertive, or to stay present during a hard conversation. Take a breath or two, and then shift your focus to your feet. How do they feel? Warm? Cool? Sore? Is the ground hard or soft? Are your shoes or socks comfortable or uncomfortable?

3. **Generate compassion.** This is a great practice for when you are feeling judgmental toward others (and even yourself) or are in need of some lighter and kinder feelings.

   In this practice, the idea is to think about the people you love and to wish them peace and kindness. Next shift to a neutral acquaintance and wish for them the same. Then shift to include yourself in the practice, and finally, to consider someone you are in conflict with. The point of this practice is that you can either stay in a state of frustration, anger, or unhappiness, or you can be in a state of wishing well for yourself and others. And generally, when we do, we feel better.

What's the Deal With Yoga?

As mind-body practices become better researched and understood, yoga and yogic practices are often done alongside other therapeutic measures. Plenty of research shows that yoga has emotional benefits along with the many physical benefits of movement.

There are many forms of yoga, and plenty of teachers with their own styles and personalities. On top of that, the classes offered might vary. There is Ashtanga, which is more rigid and systematic, and better for building discipline and strength. There is Vinyasa, which is the more "classic" type of yoga that you're more likely to walk into if you go to a studio. It is often thought of as linking breath to movement, and you'll find yourself in various poses throughout the class. Restorative or yin yoga features little movement—often, you will hold a pose with the support of blocks, blankets, bolsters, and the like to access the deepest layers of muscle and connective tissue while accessing a space of inner calm. Power yoga is more fitness-based and what you're more likely to find at a local gym—it may feature loud and energizing music and a more rigorous set of poses.

If you're depressed or down, a more active type of yoga may be most helpful. If you are anxious or trying to calm your nervous system, a slower form or restorative/yin yoga class could be supportive. But feel free to do your own research to see what might work best for you. And try out different teachers if you don't connect with the first one you try.

If you have ongoing posttraumatic stress disorder (PTSD) or have experienced sexual violence, look into trauma-informed yoga classes before walking into your local yoga studio on a whim. Many yoga teacher training programs only briefly touch upon trauma, so chances are, a random class may not offer the sort of environment that makes you feel safe or that will allow you to access your body's physical sensations with more presence.

In addition to yoga, many other mind-body practices from martial arts to qi-gong or dance can be healing, helpful, and healthy. Plus, you can even get physical education credit for some of these as well.

How Do I Manage Safety and Security Needs?

Fundamentally, do you feel safe on campus or in your living situation off campus? For some students, the question is about whether you feel safe when you're back home. Trauma and anxiety may impact your sense of safety. Do you have the accommodations that you need? How is your physical health? Do academics feel secure or tenuous? How about your friendships? Making sure you are in touch with professors, resident advisors (RAs), advisors, deans, financial aid, and whoever else you need to be in touch with, in addition to your mental health support, is a part of this, too. What do you need to do to augment your safety and security needs? Have you been able to set boundaries with roommates, not perfectly, but well enough around sleep and quiet time? Are you respecting each other's space and belongings? Are you sharing food (or not) and respecting any allergies? Try to be as specific as you can in the housing selection process. For instance, you may not want to live in a co-ed dorm, or you might want to consider a sober living dorm, if those will give you a greater sense of safety and security.

Safety and security also mean predictability. Do you have a routine? It doesn't have to be a rigid schedule, but do you make time for those things that matter? How about social time and alone time? Do you have regular times that you eat, study, and see people so that life feels predictable in a time that's often very unpredictable? Especially if you have mental health issues or executive functioning challenges, establishing routines and structure makes a difference. We know every day looks different, so we don't recommend that you make a rigid schedule such as 9:00 breakfast, 9:30 gym, 10:15 library, and so on every day, but do think in terms of *routines*—first breakfast, then exercise, then library—because this can work really well to keep some rhythm and predictability to your college life.

Many experts we spoke with reminded us of the huge shift from high school where almost every minute or hour of your day is planned, predictable, and largely managed by adults, to college, where there is so little structure and not necessarily someone to check in to make sure you're doing everything.

It can be difficult to stay organized and on top of academics, self-care, eating, and the like largely due to conflicting desires—how are you supposed to read a boring book about constitutional law when your friends are hanging out? How do you get up early to exercise before class when you participated in some event the night before? If you get FOMO (or fear of missing out), you might have to accept the MO (or missing out) part. You will almost always be missing out on something because there are often endless opportunities for things that are more fun going on. But remember to not miss out on caring for yourself, your health, your mental health, and your studies. Learning to set boundaries with yourself and others might be hard. It's not impossible to learn, but it might take some practice.

Consider your approximate daily and weekly routine. When could you study? When do you tend to socialize? When do you need to get back to your room to get ready to sleep? When do you have time to exercise? When do you go to your extracurriculars? How many classes can you realistically take, and what are reasonable goals for yourself around your grades, especially in your first year? Many schools have pass/fail options; are there some classes where that may make the most sense to give you some ease? How much time can be social before it impacts your academics, and vice versa? Maybe most crucially, you might want to set some personal boundaries with how much time you spend on social media, which can be a true time suck, negatively impact your ability to focus, and cause self-esteem issues. Research shows that the average college student spends 4.5 hours per day on social media apps. You might want to try to set up a time limit on your phone or computer for screen time usage, set up incentives (i.e., you can only look at social media for 5 minutes every 35 minutes that you get work done), or make it time- or space-based (i.e., you can look at social media between classes and at meals, or no scrolling in bed to avoid the endless pre-bedtime scroll that keeps you up until 2 a.m.).

Another challenging boundary for many students is financial. While you might've been from a similar financial background as other students in high school, in college, particularly at private schools, you might notice some extremes that can create awkwardness around casual invitations to meals, or all the suitemates splitting the expenses of a party and so forth. This might make you feel left out or less than, and eventually you might find yourself in debt to keep up. Some credit card companies prey on college students because they assume you won't read the fine print. Be sure that you are 100% clear on what you're signing up for before you commit, especially if it sounds too good to be true. And if you have a job or work-study position, you may have to think about how you schedule your hours for that to balance your work, schoolwork, and social life. Try to create a budget for yourself and stick to it.

Don't forget to create a sense of safety and security in your own room. Jasmine, a student who was miserable with homesickness, came to the counseling center to work with Chris about six weeks into school at Tufts. She was isolating in her room, hadn't unpacked her bags, and didn't decorate her room. Part of the work was just helping her feel at home by unpacking and getting her room set up.

Deb Dana, a renowned trauma therapist, talks about "triggers," the people, places, and things that activate strong negative reactions. But she also talks about the importance of creating "glimmers," the opposite of triggers—the people, places, and things that remind us that we are loved, connected, and safe. What glimmers can you create or find on campus?

Another challenge can be the lack of personal space, so we also suggest finding your own corner of campus that feels like it's your home away from your room. Maybe it's a bench on a quiet corner of campus, a particular nook in the library, or a local coffee shop.

What About Love and Belonging?

A significant predictor of success in life is the quality of our relationships and our sense of belonging. Strong relationships, even if it's just a few, directly correlate with health, mental health, and academic performance. Fortunately, you don't need hundreds of friends or to be a campus celebrity to benefit from social interaction.

So who are the people you can count on? Of course, there are the mental health experts, but over time, you will know who else to share your emotional self with, as well as who's fun to be around, great to study with, a good collaborator for social organizations, and so on. After high school, there are new opportunities for different kinds of friendships. Not every friendship has to be everything, and we caution you against only having one or two people you depend on. Different people can fill different roles in your life. And you may not want or need to (or maybe even shouldn't) share your mental health challenges with everyone. As long as you have a few people who know your struggles and your strengths, and can be relied upon if you need more vulnerable support, that's good enough.

Where do you belong? Where can you try to connect, and who can help you connect if that's a struggle for you? Are you making enough time for social connection? Develop and tend to relationships with the people who inspire you to be more yourself and the version of yourself that you want to become. And we don't mean just with other students—be sure to have some "adults" in your corner on campus, too. Are there any professors or staff you really admire, or some other adult on campus who inspires you? Forge that relationship by going to office hours or emailing them to get a coffee.

What Are Esteem Needs?

Maslow describes the idea of self-esteem as feeling a sense of dignity, achievement, and independence, as well as the acceptance, respect, and support of our peers. Who are the people who see you and respect you, who truly bring you up? Who are those people? Do they make you feel good about yourself or add to feelings of inadequacy?

Try This: Write down the names of a few people who believe in you, who make you feel good about yourself, and who you can trust. Write down the names of a few people who bring you down, who make you feel small and insignificant. Next, write down how much time you spend with each and reflect on your answers.

Do you take a sense of pride in your school and your schoolwork? What about your leadership in clubs, activities, and teams? What have been your successes? What are the things that you're good at? Are those the things you are doing for yourself, or have you joined clubs or taken academic courses to satisfy or impress other people? Most importantly, which aspects of yourself can you take pride in that aren't based on what you do or your achievements, but who you are? Keep track of these for those moments when you are feeling down to remind yourself of how incredible you truly are.

A friend once said, "If you want self-esteem, perform esteemable acts." What are those things in your life? The poet Yung Pueblo, also known as Diego Perez, reminds us to try to find three daily wins: a physical win like exercise or movement; a mental win like reading, writing, learning, or creating; and a spiritual win like connecting to or helping others, or spending time in nature, praying, or meditating. What are your three daily wins today? Perhaps spend a week or two trying this out each night before you go to bed and see how it feels.

What Is Actualization?

Actualization is the process of becoming your best self, in line with your values. Leaving home is an excellent time to reflect on who you want to be and how to live in accordance with your values. What are your values? One way to answer this question is to ask yourself how you would want to be remembered by your friends and classmates.

Beyond school, do you take a sense of esteem from your home community, culture, spiritual practice, or other aspects of your identity? What are your other joys, your hobbies, interest in arts, and different sports? These, too, can fulfill our need for actualization. Finding authentic meaning and purpose will bring you closer to actualization as well. One of the best ways you can do that is to research through acts of community service, volunteering, and the generosity of helping others. In doing so, we quickly get out of our own heads when we make a deliberate effort to help others. Maybe that's volunteering with local kids as a tutor or basketball coach, doing work through a campus activist or community service group, or getting off campus to engage with the local community. And here's another idea: Consider taking a year off to find yourself.

I took a year off when I was depressed my junior year. I had no idea what to do with myself in that time, but my parents made me volunteer at my old elementary school where my aunt worked. I actually discovered I loved working with kids, and now coach kids' basketball and am working on my degree to be a children's librarian.

—Kai, working on a master's degree in library science

Still, we can't overemphasize the importance of self-care. You are optimizing the likelihood that you will succeed.

Exercise: Write down your self-care plan, including sleep, exercise, meals, friendships, clubs, and mentors. Now write down the opposite of what you just wrote. For instance, if you wrote down "three meals a day," write down "skipping meals"; if you wrote down "fun time with friends and eight hours of sleep," write down "partying all night and getting no sleep." Look at your answers; self-care should be clear.

How Do I Manage Stress in a Nonstop Environment?

Chris once had a supervisor remind him, "Calm makes everything better; stress makes everything worse." It's true. Stress makes emotions more difficult to manage, makes us perceive everything in a negative light, and even negatively impacts our physical health. Of course, a small amount of stress is okay and is just evolution's way of having us deal with a novel situation. We all get stressed, but you can avoid it spiraling out of control by knowing what your stress red flags are (see p. 142 in this chapter for a checklist).

What are the signs of stress for you? Consider the physical, the mental, the interpersonal, and the behavioral. Some of us go into fight mode and get aggressive, irritable, anxious, or avoidant; some of us go into freeze and feel paralyzed; others of us go into fuck it mode and just give up.

We want you to think up some ways you can manage stress when you see it coming. It might be helpful to even consider what you might do or suggest for a friend and do it for yourself. But we also have a few ideas.

For one thing, it helps to "name and tame" and recognize that you are stressed; let yourself label this as stress, and then it becomes more manageable. Try some breathing practices, like the 7–11 breath. For this one, you breathe in through your nostrils as you count to seven, and out through your mouth as you count to eleven. This gets you out of the fight or flight response. Alternately, if you're in the freeze or fuck-it response, reverse the ratio. In fact, breathing in longer and out shorter can help you focus if your mind is wandering, or you're feeling tired or sluggish. Slowing the breath like this settles the nervous system and even redirects blood flow to the parts of the brain associated with emotional regulation.

You can also try self-compassion exercises, like giving yourself a hug, or placing a hand over your heart. This gentle touch appears to quiet the stress response as well, slowing down the release of cortisol, just like getting a hug from a friend. And if you're struggling to sleep or feel settled in your body, try the progressive muscle relaxation exercise below, called the CALM reminder, popularized by Herbert Benson.

The CALM Reminder

Allow your eyes to close, and your body to relax. Take a few extended breaths and then begin the exercise.

C–Chest

*After a few breaths, bring your awareness into your **chest** and torso area. First scan your chest, and allow lungs and belly to fully expand with the breath. Notice any sensations there.*

Is your breath shallow and short, or slow and even? Is your heart beating quickly or slowly? Is there any tightness or tension in your chest? Tension or relaxation?
Now, tense all the muscles throughout your chest and torso, and hold for a count of three as you feel the tension, then allow your muscles to relax. Feel the tension to flow away, and the relaxation to flow in through the next few breaths.

A–Arms

*Now shift your attention to your **arms**, from your shoulders down to the tips of your fingers. Are your hands hot and sweaty? Cold and clammy? Shaking or still? Can you just allow them to settle if they are shaking?*

Now, squeeze your fists, tense your arms all the way up to your shoulders and hold for three breaths, feeling any physical and emotional tension, then let go and let your arms relax completely. Enjoy three more breaths, enjoying the newfound relaxation flow into your arms.

L–Legs

*On the next breath, direct your attention down to your **legs**, from your hips down through your toes. Notice if your legs are communicating anything in this moment, sometimes they bounce with anxiety or stress, and then just allow them to become still.*

Now, gently squeeze the muscles in your feet, then up through your legs and waist, holding that tension for three breaths, and then release. Take three more breaths as you feel the tension flowing out of your legs, and just offer your legs some thanks for the work they do. Maybe even practice gratitude for all the work they do all day!

M–Mouth

*Last, bring your attention to your **mouth** and jaw, where many of us hold emotional tension and stress.*

Which emotion is your mouth expressing inwardly and outwardly—stress, anxiety, anger? Something else? Finally, clench your mouth and jaw, holding for three breaths, and then release.

After this brief practice, notice your state of tension or relaxation. If it helps, do it on days that you feel particularly stressed or before going to bed at night. It's hard to have a stressed mind and a relaxed body at the same time, and by relaxing your body, you relax your mind, so use the CALM reminder whenever you need some relaxation.

HALT Check-In

It can take a lot of self-awareness to notice increasing stress; however, there is an acronym that helps, and you can check in with yourself every day. Are you:

H–Hungry?
A–Angry/Anxious?
L–Lonely?
T–Tired?

If any of these apply, can you:

1. Get something to eat?
2. Do the breathing exercises we just reviewed to lower your anger or anxiety?
3. Reach out to a friend or sit in a public place so you're around other people?
4. Take a nap, adjust your sleep schedule, or change your sleeping arrangements?

There are four foundations to resilience. First, you need to get a good night's sleep as that will affect quality of life. Second, eat a healthy diet, which may seem obvious but can be a challenge for an emerging adult. Third, be physically active. This can be any beneficial movement. It doesn't need to be a strenuous workout class, but getting up and about, like taking a walk or stretching. This also encourages a change of scenery, which is good for the brain. Fourth, cultivate quality social support. I gently inquire with students on how they are doing in these well-being categories. Many stressed students come for counseling, and we assess that they are not getting sleep, they are skipping meals, are holed up in a library or dorm room, are worried about fitting in and friendships, and may be lonely. So we can start with these basics first because this is how students can resource themselves.

—**Dr. Tara Cousineau, Harvard College staff clinician**

Dr. Cousineau also talks about learning to manage our own nervous systems. When we're stressed, the body often goes into a fight or flight reaction. This is natural and part of the base operating system of being a human. But over time this can lead to burnout, and students with chronic stress, and who may lack coping skills, can fall into freeze and faint responses because life feels so overwhelming. Sometimes there are traumatic situations as well. Where students typically get stuck is that they disconnect from their bodies. They start in their head, especially if they are intellectual by nature. You may find a personal reason for your stress, "I'm not good enough, smart enough, attractive enough, or whatever enough." That's a "top down" approach and it fuels your inner critic. But often it makes more sense to start from the "bottom up" and tend to the body, such as the physical manifestations of stress, and begin to regulate your autonomic nervous system. This in turn allows some stability to then address your stress triggers and accompanying emotions and thoughts.

When you're in fight/flight mode, or feel activated by anxiety and anger, often you need to reach a place of calm and connection, such as relaxation, breathwork, meditation, have a long shower or bath, listen to soothing or quiet music, and generally slow down. On the other hand, if you're in more of a shut down or freeze/faint response, you may need to energize yourself. For example, practicing activating breathwork (e.g., bellow breath), engaging in physical movement, listening to energizing music, and even eating spicy foods. This can help speed things up a bit and shift you into a more regulated and connected place.

What Are Some Other Self-Care and Self-Soothing Activities?

Many of the following ideas may seem obvious, but we often forget the power of everyday activities. For instance, if you are reading this and feeling stressed right now, try any of these with the intention of noticing what happens to stress:

1. Take a shower.
2. Write about your day.
3. Write down your worries.
4. Go for a walk.
5. Watch a movie or show that'll make you laugh.
6. Play a game.
7. Lie down on grass in a park or the quad.
8. Get off campus (maybe take a friend).

Are none of those sounding good right now? What other activities could you do? Try that. Once you do an activity, write down how the activity impacted your stress.

Sometimes we need a whole "mental health day." If you take a mental health day, we encourage you to actively take care of yourself that day and change your environment. Go home or off campus if you can do so. Visit a museum, see a movie, have a spa day, or go to the gym or a fitness class. And reach out: Have a long phone call or Facetime with a friend or sibling, or make a plan to meet up with someone that day (or take them with you). One thing we do not recommend for a mental health day is more isolating (unless you're experiencing social burnout) because human contact is important for managing our stress and not just bouncing around in our own heads.

But just a word of caution: Doing any activity to reduce stress is key if the focus is on reducing stress. However, don't use stress reduction activities as avoidance. If you do, avoidance will feel good in the moment but cause you much more stress in the long run. You have to be honest with yourself. Avoidance has the quality of constantly procrastinating, whereas stress reduction is reducing your level of stress in order to get to what you need to do.

Time Management and Other Campus Resources

Whether or not you have an executive function diagnosis, time management can be very difficult. In high school, classes were scheduled throughout the day and held within a relatively small campus. In college, classes are not as regularly scheduled, and the campuses tend to be much larger. Many schools have faculty who can help you with organizational skills and practices, and many of these resources are available through the resource or counseling centers.

If you are someone who tends to be organized, you might not need to see someone to help you, but nevertheless, a calendar, agenda, or whiteboard in your room can help you be even more organized. Use it to note not just your classes, office hours, and appointments, but block out time to exercise, eat meals, see friends, and do self-care activities. This is especially important during more stressful times like midterms or finals!

Find Perspective

Stress distorts priorities and perspective. It might help to remember past times you've felt stress and the healthy ways you've gotten through it. Or even simply the fact that you got through it at all! It may help to remember also that this moment will eventually pass, just like the others did.

If you are willing to get silly, the practice of laughter is a great way to destress. If you want, simply start laughing. Alternatively, watch a standup routine, join an improv group, listen to a funny podcast, or read a funny book. Laughter not only keeps your brain creative, but it causes the release of serotonin, the brain chemical associated with joy.

Or can you lean on your culture or faith? Which rituals, beliefs, and traditions can help you through hard times? Which aspects of your culture can keep you grounded?

Shift Your Focus

Dr. Cousineau from Harvard also suggests "get a three minute sand timer—or use a mobile phone timer—and focus on your feet or your breath for three minutes. Ground your body. See what happens. Or, focus on your body sensations for three minutes. Where am I feeling tension or constriction? Then direct kind awareness to that area. You can even place a hand over the heart, or fold arms across the torso, and be still. Simple physical gestures can change how you feel. Often, the intense feelings will fade by the end of the three minutes and you are ready to have a conversation."

Campus is a bubble, and sometimes just stepping off campus into the town or city can put things into perspective. It can be easy to get caught up in all of the happenings (and sometimes drama) that occur in that specific area. Find some nearby hiking trails or get out in nature. Take the bus into the city and check out the museums, shops, restaurants, cafes, and cultural attractions. If you find that this reduces stress, make a point of going off campus more often. Add these to your calendar. You could even make a bucket list of all the local things you'd like to do before you graduate and make your way through it over the years.

Now that you've read this section, write down the elements that resonate with you and commit to do these. Ideally, you would have a friend who you could do things with and could help keep you accountable to your commitment to self-care.

How Do I Handle Setbacks When They Emerge?

Very few students cruise through college without some bumps in the road, and this is particularly true for those who struggle with mental health challenges. Setbacks should be expected. No matter how hard you plan, you can never anticipate everything that could happen. When you are in the thick of it, it may feel on the outside as if everyone is just cruising on by socially, academically, emotionally, and more. Remember: Don't compare how you feel on the inside to how other people look on the outside. Especially on social media!

So what can you do when you hit the inevitable setback? Here are some ideas:

How Can I Make a Coping Plan?

The Cope Ahead Plan comes from DBT (read more on Chapters 4 and 6). It's the practice of imagining the worst-case scenario and then planning for what you'll do should that worst thing happen. For example, say you have to give a presentation for one of your classes. Now, let's say that you are well rehearsed, but you worry that you will freeze in the moment. Your Cope Ahead Plan would be for freezing, if that is your worst worry. By preparing for such an eventuality, you increase your chance of dealing with a potential setback. In effect, you are coping ahead if it happens. Let's break it down:

1. Start by writing down the situation that may lead to uncomfortable emotions. For example, "I have to give a talk on: 'Should supreme executive power derive from a mandate from the masses, or is it a divine right?' The talk is next Tuesday and will take place in front of 20 classmates."
2. Next, name the emotions or other concerns that might show up and get in the way of you doing your best presentation.
3. Decide which specific coping skills you want to use in the situation. Does slowing your breath help? Is there a medication like a beta blocker that you sometimes take for this type of anxiety? Does drinking coffee help or hurt? Will having a supportive classmate in the front row help you relax? What else could work for you?
4. Vividly imagine the situation. Visualize the environment as realistically as possible. Imagine standing in front of the class. How does the room smell? What do you see? Use all of your senses as you envision this moment. (Maybe you want to even go to the classroom when it's empty to make it feel even more real!)
5. Next, as you imagine that situation, rehearse in your mind coping effectively and the exact steps you'll take. From the start of your presentation, rehearse your talk, what you will say, and how you will say it, and practice how you'll cope if it gets tough. Are there any other problems that might arise? Ideally, by coping ahead with the challenge, anything that arises should be easier to deal with in the moment.
6. Once you've completed the exercise, give yourself some self-care afterward. This exercise can be a lot!

How Can I Change My Mindset and Perspective?

Often the thing that holds us back is the fear of failure. This kind of worry is very common in college. By holding onto the fear that you might fail, it may feel impossible to start and lead to avoidance. Maybe you worry about handing in the term paper you've already finished because you think it's not good enough and that your professor is going to be disappointed, so you avoid handing it in and going to class. If this sounds like you, try some of these tips:

1. **Actively challenge your assumptions**. With the term paper example, are you assuming that you will do badly? Are you assuming that your professor will judge it poorly? Challenge the assumptions by labeling assumptions as assumptions, and facts as facts.

   I have a paper due Tuesday (fact).

   It is on "The Nature of Light" (fact).

   I am going to fail this paper (assumption).

   My professor is going to think that I'm stupid (assumption).

   In this case, think about the things that are in your control. If you're worried that your work isn't up to par, does the professor have office hours to go over your concerns with you, or is there a teaching assistant who could help?

2. **Reflect on and evaluate the current situation**. If you're worried about failing, it can help to assess the situation on your own or with someone you trust. For example, you could ask yourself: "Am I failing this course? Will this paper make or break my grade? If I don't do as well as I want to, does that make me a failure? Are there things that I can do to improve my grade if it doesn't go well?" Of course, in some situations, it may actually be that bad, but in many, you might be turning a molehill setback into a mountain. Separate the possible setback from who you are. You are not a failure, and setbacks don't define you. Your thoughts are just thoughts, and you don't have to believe them all. You are having the thought that you will fail, which doesn't mean that you will.

3. **Expand your timeline**. There is fascinating research on how our emotions change our perception of time (Droit-Volet, 2007).[2] The phenomenon is known as the time-emotion paradox. For example, the passage of time seems to fluctuate depending on whether you are in a pleasant or unpleasant situation. When you are spending time with a love interest at dinner, time seems to fly by; however, waiting to meet with your professor to discuss your term paper can feel interminable. Now that you know that we are so wrong in estimating time when we experience strong emotions, you can challenge yourself to change your perception of time in this scenario. If you are worried about failing the course because of a paper, remember the emotion is making you feel like the moment will last for a long time. Will a poor grade matter in five days? How might I feel about it in five weeks, months, or years? (As Chris's children's book tells us, "Feelings are like farts—they linger, but

never last." It'll pass.) More practically, do you have enough time now to get the help you need, or to even take one last look over it before you submit it?

Other similar research reminds us to think through beyond the worst-case scenario: "So I fail the test, what will I do next? Okay, I'll cry, I'll feel sorry for myself for a while, but eventually I'll get my laundry done, eat dinner, and hang out with friends." Expand the timeline beyond just the bad moment and the immediate aftermath.

Reflect on Past Wins

Write down past setbacks or "failures" and reflect on what strengths or skills you leaned on to overcome those situations. Some of the answers may seem trivial and some may seem big, but they all count. We all learn from difficult moments, so what is the lesson? For instance, maybe previously you had difficulty asking for help, but then you learned that it's okay and normal to ask for help when you need it, and that your friends will have your back when things don't go as planned. Maybe you lost a friendship because you had to set boundaries, but you felt more peaceful because you didn't have that person in your life anymore and learned to stand up for yourself. What are you experiencing currently, and what can you learn from it?

Bouncing back from setbacks is never an easy process, and we don't mean to make it sound like it is. And yet you would not have gotten this far without overcoming some setbacks in the past, so we encourage you to let yourself be your own inspiration as you make your way through this one. We hope that these tools make it a bit easier on you going forward!

You might even want to write them down and reflect on what you did to overcome those situations. Some of the answers you come up with may seem trivial and some may seem big, but they all count. We learn from difficult moments. What have you learned? For instance, maybe previously you had difficulty in asking for help, but then maybe you found out that asking for help was not such a scary proposition. You may have learned that it's okay to ask for help when you need it or that your friends will have your back when things don't go as planned.

EXERCISE: What is a situation now that feels like a setback?

What or who has helped me overcome other setbacks in the past?

Is there anyone I can reach out to whom I trust?

Do I know what resources are available on campus? When are office hours?

How Can I Get Better at Difficult Things?

The best way to get better at hard things is to practice! Ultimately, your job is to go after the things you want most, even if you are afraid. Like the old self-help books say, feel the fear and do it anyway! Start with hard things that are low stakes. Then, two things will happen: The first is that you'll know that you can do them, and the second is that they might actually be fun.

If you are embarrassed by your dance moves, can you join a dance club or take a local class? If you fear public speaking, can you join a public speaking class or improv group? And when it comes to public performances like those, a trick is to try to convince yourself that what you're feeling in your body (heart pounding, palms sweating, etc.) is not just fear, but maybe excitement. It might feel difficult and awkward at first, but it will become easier. Stretching your comfort zone and creativity is one of the best ways to bring about new ideas and perspectives on school, on friendships, and on challenging emotional situations, too.

EXERCISE: What is one activity *just* outside of my comfort zone that may be fun to do?

How Do I Recognize My Red Flags?

Our hope is that this section provides you with some clear, objective measures to have an honest check-in with yourself. Then you'll know when it's time to seek support, ramp up self-care practices, or make other changes to stay balanced and on track for what you need to do.

Red Flags Checklist

Self-Care

- ☐ Have you taken a shower and brushed your teeth in the past 24 hours?
- ☐ When's the last time you did something for your own enjoyment?
- ☐ Are you eating enough every day?

☐ Are you sleeping regularly, at least as much as a college student can?

☐ Are you drinking enough fluids every day?

☐ How much are you indulging in alcohol or using substances? Quantify your use.

☐ Are you drinking alcohol or using substances on your own or with others? How often for each scenario?

☐ Are you managing to keep your room relatively clean?

☐ Have you been seeing your doctor/therapist/other medical provider?

☐ Are you taking your medication as prescribed?

☐ Are you setting good boundaries with work/life/fun balance?

Academics

☐ Are you behind or avoiding any assignments?

☐ Have you been getting to class? Is there a class that you're avoiding? If so, why?

Work/Internship

☐ Do you regularly go to your job/internship?

☐ Have you been searching for internships/jobs and making summer and postgraduation plans?

Clubs/Organizations/Athletics

☐ Have you been fulfilling your roles in clubs and activities?

☐ Do you show up to practice and games if you're an athlete?

☐ Are you able to balance everything required for your club/organization/sport and your academic, social, work/internship, and self-care needs or responsibilities?

Relationships: Social

☐ Have you been seeing friends? Have you been isolating?

☐ Have you been getting involved with some groups or organizations on campus?

☐ Are you avoiding doing other things that you need or want to do in favor of your social life?

☐ Do you demand that your friends meet your needs?

Relationships: Romantic

☐ Are you enjoying the time you spend with the person you're seeing?

☐ Are you ignoring any ways that your feelings are hurt by the romantic situation that you're in?

☐ Are you avoiding getting other things done (i.e., school work, internship applications, work, self-care, etc.) in order to spend time with the person you're seeing?

☐ Do you expect your romantic interest to meet all of your needs?

Now that you've gone through this check-in, we suggest doing either the journaling or the meditation exercise (or both!), and then the small action exercise. These will help you process what you learned or reflected on here, ground yourself, and then make some moves toward what you're needing right now.

Journaling Exercise

Write down what you noticed. Are there any patterns? Is there one section where you are having more trouble or experiencing more stress? Is there anything that you've been avoiding more than the other things that you indicated? Is there anything that you feel more capable of doing now that you look at it?

After writing it out, how are you feeling? Does it feel any better to get it out and notice what's been weighing on you? How's your stress level in this moment? What feels most pressing to address after completing this journal exercise?

Feeling Stuck?

Try This: Take one small thing. What is one seemingly small thing that you can do right now to meet this need? If you have an idea, it is important that you do it. Thinking about it will typically keep you stuck in a cycle of thinking about it (not fun). So go. Send that email to your professor! Send that text to your friend! Make that call to the therapist you've been meaning to connect with! Go for a quick walk outside and leave your room! Clean your room for five minutes while listening to your favorite song! Drink a glass of water! Take a shower! Eat a snack! Go and do it now. We know that some of these don't necessarily feel small. Just keep it to something that can be done in no more than 20 minutes. Ideally, even just five minutes should be sufficient.

Checking In: Did you do it? Take a moment to recognize your accomplishment. Doesn't feel like one? It is, especially when doing it is difficult for you. Don't take one thing that you do for granted, especially if things have been tough and you've found yourself unable to take action. Any healthy move, consistent with your goals and values, should be celebrated.

Feeling Down?

Try This: The Self-Compassion Break.[3] These ideas come from the work of Drs. Chris Germer and Kristen Neff, both of whom are experts in self-compassion:

> Find a comfortable seat. Close your eyes, or focus on a spot just in front of you. Put one hand on your heart and the other hand on your belly. Take a big inhale through your nostrils, allowing the air to go down to your belly, noticing it expand under your hand. When you exhale, see if you can exhale through your mouth as slowly as you can, either sighing it out, or blowing the air out with "blowfish" lips a few times.

> Rest for a few moments and just notice how your body, heart, and mind feel now. Which physical sensations are you experiencing? How do you feel emotionally? What are your current thoughts as you do this practice?

> Now bring to mind a difficult recent situation, and start with something relatively easy to deal with like running late for class, forgetting something, procrastinating, or a small mistake you made recently. Do you notice a critical inner voice?

> Now just validate yourself with a few kind words, the ones you might use with a friend. "This is hard, this sucks, this is painful." Or whatever feels authentic to you.

> Notice if anything changes. If it does, note that; if nothing changes, note that as well.

> Now give yourself a hug or place a hand over your heart, and again notice if there's a shift. Try offering yourself some words that remind you that you're not alone. "College is tough, nobody's perfect, we all make mistakes, everyone on campus is stressed or gets overwhelmed sometimes." Just pick words and a tone that feel like those you'd want to share, or you'd want to hear from a friend.

> Lastly, make a wish for yourself, again like you'd offer a friend. "May I let this go, may I forgive myself . . . may I learn from this, may I move on . . ." Try a few phrases until you settle on whatever words feel right to you.

> Allow a few moments for the words to sink in, as well as the warm sensations of your hands on your heart or giving yourself a hug.

Now open your eyes or raise them and look around your space. Let your eyes rest on an object that makes you feel happy or smile. Maybe a picture with your friends or a gift from your family. Notice how that object makes you feel for around 30 seconds. What's happening in your body? What's happening emotionally? Have your thoughts changed?

How Can I Get Involved in Mental Health Activism?

Once you are more effective and skilled at taking care of yourself, you might want to give back and help others who are feeling hopeless. And sometimes it can help us find a sense of meaning, a feeling of presence, or feel connected to our purpose when we give to others. Feel out of control? Try to control what you can. Feel helpless? Try helping others! Feel disempowered? Get active and start making change on campus and beyond. Research finds that activism and service are some of the best ways to feel like we are making the world a better place, boost our mood, and enhance our sense of agency and purpose when we have struggled with trauma and mental illness.

You may want to get involved with mental health activism as you go through the process of taking care of yourself and getting support. Maybe everything you've been going through could be used to help someone else feel understood or to experience a kinder world than you have.

What Can I Do to Get Involved?

Join a mental health activism organization or club. Look into your options on campus, and in your local community. Is there a group with a meeting coming up? Go! Maybe there is an Active Minds chapter that you can get involved with—Active Minds is a young adult–oriented mental health support group. There is also the National Alliance on Mental Illness (NAMI) on Campus, the Jed Foundation, Mental Health America, the Trevor Project, the Black Mental Health Alliance, UROK, Youth Move, Higher Education Mental Health Alliance, Students Against Depression, International Conference of Young People in Alcoholics Anonymous (ICYPAA), and more.

Start your own. Don't have or don't like the options on campus or locally? DIY! If you have the interest and some extra time, put it together. What do you want the focus to be—a specific mental health issue or something more general? Do you want to put on events, engage in advocacy efforts on campus or beyond, create zines, start a helpline, or something else? Who else could join? Get to brainstorming and follow your excitement, goals, and values!

Have brave conversations. Some of the best activism we can do is embedded into our everyday experiences. If someone says or does something that shows that they might be lacking awareness around mental health issues, see if you can bring yourself to say something. Sometimes just engaging with the person with an open mind and curiosity makes for an ideal environment for you to help them understand. Of course, honor your capacity for this—if you're not feeling so up to it, that's okay. If this is someone who you can be in touch with later when you have the capacity, you can always share with them or send some resources then.

Advocate for better mental health support on campus. Maybe through your experience you've found a way that others in your position could be better supported. Not enough therapists on campus, or enough diversity in the options for therapists in the counseling center? Is there a climate of silence and stigma in your fraternity or sorority? Have you experienced microaggressions? See if the offices or staff members involved are willing to hear you out—maybe they can help make those changes. And if not, you can always try to spread awareness of the issue on social media, with posters, letters, or larger actions to get your college's attention. Run for student government or write letters to the board of trustees—there's a lot of concrete action you can take to create change, especially when you have a team of other activists, too.

In Conclusion

Self-care can be hard work. It's not just bubble baths and massages—it's an active and daily commitment to keeping yourself healthy and growing. And it's not selfish. Taking good care of yourself allows you to be there for others because it increases your capacity to engage more fully, and with greater care and patience. And it doesn't have to be done by yourself! Relationships are a key part of self-care, and they also can motivate us to get to that yoga class, cook that healthy meal, or try that new community service club we feel a bit shy about going to on our own.

Chapter 7
Supporting Others

You may have picked up this book not just for yourself, but maybe because you're a student leader or resident advisor (RA), or even a faculty, family, or friend to someone dealing with mental health issues. You may also want to read this chapter if you yourself are having a mental health episode or to think about what kind of support to ask of others.

A word of caution: Although we obviously have excellent advice in this book, reading it from cover to cover will not qualify you as mental health professional, no matter what degree you are working on! If you are hungry for more, that may be a sign that you could be an excellent candidate to work in mental health. As an old therapist told Chris before he embarked on graduate school: "There are some people who need therapy once a week, and then those unfortunates who need it twice a week. Then there are people like you and me, who need forty hours a week of therapy. I think this is your calling, Chris."

But one of the most important things to remember when supporting others is to take good care of yourself. The people in your life who you wish to support need a well-rested, healthy, and *not* burned-out support network, so self-care, along with knowing your limits and boundaries, will be key. If you are getting burned out, feeling out of your element, losing sight of your boundaries, or feeling helpless, a mental health professional needs to step in. In fact, even professionals are ethically required to step back and get help when we're experiencing those things. The reality is that despite your best intentions, your advice could do more harm than good. For example, if someone is experiencing psychosis and hearing voices, recommending a good night's sleep and ignoring the voices may be well-intentioned advice but is actually a condition that needs medication and professional care, so your recommendation would not be helpful. Still, for many students, their experience does not rise to the most challenging of experiences, and there are many things that you can do to help someone who's just having a tough day.

How Can I Support a Friend, Family Member, or Student Who Is Struggling?

Being supportive isn't always easy. After all, you have all your own stuff going on between school, work, family and friends, and who knows what else. And we typically tend to offer advice from our own point of view and struggle with knowing what the "right" thing to say is.

If there is one skill we want to share, it is validation. Validation is a technique to show empathy toward what someone is going through. By validating, you create a supportive and nonjudgmental environment, like a therapist. We simply recognize that a person's experience is valid and remain curious and open to their perspective. You might not agree with their reactions to things, or even understand it, but you are showing that you believe them, that their experiences matter to you and are real.

Here's a concrete example. Your friend says that she is hungry, and you make her a peanut butter sandwich. She rejects it. You could get judgmental and tell her that peanut butter is delicious and that you went out of your way to make the sandwich and that she is an ungrateful person. But instead, you want to validate and get curious. She tells you that she is allergic to peanuts and got anxious when you brought the sandwich into the room, because not only would it not help her if she was hungry but was even dangerous. By validating her experience, you understand more, you get closer to her, she feels heard by you, the relationship strengthens, and as a bonus, a helpful solution is likely to emerge. Validation does *not* mean that you have to agree that peanut butter is bad or good; it just means that a person's experience and reactions are legit.

Validation acknowledges your friend's experience without judgment, criticism, trying to change how they see things, or even fixing it. Again, you don't have to agree with or condone their behavior. In the above example, say that you are a vegetarian and they are a carnivore, and they want a ham sandwich. If you're a vegetarian for religious or ethical issues, this does not mean that you now condone the eating of animals, just because she does. It also means that given who your friend is, with her allergies and preferences, that her choices are valid and understandable.

Now, hunger is one thing. Emotional struggles are another. For example, say that your friend is upset because he broke up with his girlfriend. It was the right thing to do because she was cheating on him. In this case, you might feel strongly that it was absolutely the right move; nevertheless, it is also valid he feels sad about the breakup, because even though she was not the right person for him, she was funny, and she made him laugh. You can validate the breakup and how sad it makes him feel, because both are his experience. On the flip side, your suggestion that he start looking for a new hookup might not be helpful in the moment.

Types of Validation in Dialectical Behavioral Therapy

We love how Dialectical Behavioral Therapy (DBT) offers validation skills for peers and parents and even professors of people struggling (see Chapter 4). In fact, DBT has six levels of validation, and each can be useful for supporting a friend. Validation strengthens individuals and relationships, by helping the other person know they are not crazy or alone, even that their emotions and behaviors make sense, and that you are someone who will hear them out without judgment or criticism. Imagine having a friend like that!

Level 1—Just Being Present. How many times do we get distracted when our friends are trying to talk to us? How often are we on our phones or paying attention to something else? The first level of validation is the simple act of being completely present and attentive to your friend. You are holding or creating a safer space where they can express and unburden themselves. When a friend reaches out, depending on the urgency, your boundaries are important, too. Offer a good time, like not in the middle of studying for a final, and then when you connect, put down your devices, and just be there with them, fully present. You might even bring some mindful awareness to your breath, posture, tone, and body language to show your openness.

Level 2—Accurate Reflection. How often does someone tell us something, and then what we hear or interpret is very different from what they mean? One of us once asked a group of people learning DBT skills on Zoom what state they were in, meaning emotional state. Participants heard the question as meaning what state in the nation they were Zooming in from, and one chemistry major thought it meant state of matter—solid, liquid, or gas. Accurate reflection is the act of repeating back what you heard and making sure that you understood what the other person was saying in the way they meant it. If you're not sure, just ask someone. "It sounds like you're saying or feeling _____. Do I have that right?"

Active listening is listening with our full attention and sometimes offering subtler reflections as well. Creating and holding that space for a friend by just listening can itself be incredibly powerful and helpful for them, as well as helping settle their nervous system when you can stay calm as well. You can also acknowledge what the person is feeling, just with a few words, or those "empathic sighs" and "mm-hmms" that therapists are famous for, and sometimes really annoying with. But make sure these are genuine: No one feels better with fake empathy. These encourage the person to keep talking, maybe even coming to their own solutions. When we care about someone, we often do want to start by problem-solving and offering advice. It's a good instinct, but if the person is emotional, not a lot may get through and trying to immediately problem-solve or to give advice can hurt more than it helps. Very little is going to sink in until the person has settled and regulated their emotions, often with our help by just listening.

You can also show that you understand how they feel by just expressing a wish for them, rather than offering a solution, or even saying that their perspective is right. "Ugh, I wish that the professor was a little more flexible, too, man." "Oh sweetie, I really wish that had never happened to your friend." Just those kinds of words help people feel seen, and more importantly, feel *felt* in their emotional experience. This kind of compassionate validation can go a long way toward being supportive, and it is actually easier and often more effective than trying to solve the problem in the moment. In fact, in Chapter 6, we talked about how to offer this kind of support to ourselves too with self-compassion (see Chapter 6).

Level 3—Reading Between the Lines. People who are emotionally sensitive, often those with depression and anxiety, can be very attuned to others' emotions. Those less emotionally sensitive may have a difficult time knowing what they are feeling. Reading between the lines means noticing expressions, tone, and verbal and body language that can tell you more about what someone is feeling than they may be aware of. It may seem obvious that if someone is crying, they are sad, or that if they cringe, they might be scared. While it may feel obvious to you, it may not be obvious to them, or vice versa. This can be especially challenging across cultures and backgrounds.

If you do point out a reaction, keep it curious rather than telling them, and explain why you think that they may be feeling a certain way. For instance, "I noticed that when you were talking about the guy you went out with last night, you sighed and looked away. That made me wonder if it didn't go well."

Again, you don't actually know, you simply noticed a reaction and inferred something from the reaction, and you pointed it out, but it is up to the person to share their experience.

Level 4—Understanding Your Friend's Behavior, Given Their Experiences. This means recognizing that someone's actions and emotions are understandable and valid, given their history, experiences, biology, and other circumstances. Maybe the friend is from a community where alcohol is forbidden. It would make sense, given where they are from, their societal norms, and religious views, that they would not want to come to a kegger with you. Or, say that your friend was once bitten by a dog and needed intravenous antibiotics, they might be skeptical of bringing your dog to your apartment next semester. Again, staying curious about the other's experience will help you to see how their responses make sense.

Level 5—Acknowledging the Validity of the Person's Emotions, Given Current Circumstances. Here, you simply recognize that, given what a person is going through in this present moment, and in these current circumstances, that their emotions make sense. If your friend is worried about a sick relative, they will be distracted by the worry and more likely to fail the test. Given that your friend is struggling with bigger worries, those emotions and worries make sense. You can express empathy and support for what they are going through, even just saying, "That sounds hard." Just naming the experience, not having to get much more specific, can really help someone manage their overwhelming emotions.

When we "name to tame" the emotion, by naming the experience back to your friend, ideally in their words, you don't want to put words into their mouth, and so if you're not sure, just ask: "It sounds like you're feeling pretty pissed off right now. Is that right?" Actually naming the emotion activates the more rational parts of the brain and quiets the emotional parts of the brain, helping to calm the nervous system as well. This is what we therapists do all the time: We help people recognize what they are feeling so they can settle and work with the challenge with their whole brain, not just their emotional reaction.

Level 6—Radical Genuineness. This approach recognizes the humanity in all of us, to empathize with the suffering of others no matter what they are going through. You might cry with them, laugh with them, and be angry with them. You can be transparent about how you feel about what they are going through in an authentic and connected way. In this level, you don't even need words, because sometimes when you give someone a tissue or a hug, it lets them know that you get it.

You don't have to wonder about what level of validation you are express-ing, and we have broken these down into levels in order to give you some ideas that could be helpful. And remember, you don't have to problem-solve; often the first thing people need is just the compassionate presence of another.

Here are some key points when validating:

1. Don't offer solutions before validating, unless the person asks for them. In the case of the breakup, your roommate may not be ready to date, and they might not have gotten over their romantic partners. Start with validating how difficult this is for them, rather than saying: "They were a total jerk. Let's start swiping. I can show you this cute girl in my econ class I think you'd like." As a friend, parent, or educator, you can always just ask, "Do you want me to just listen now, or would you like me to help problem-solve a bit, too?" The harder part is to respect their answer.

2. Focus on their emotional needs before supporting them with words and thoughts. We are born as emotional beings and are emotional way before we become verbal beings. You will find that when you soothe your friend emotionally, it will be much easier to then soothe them with thoughts and words.

3. It is hard to think when you are emotionally overwhelmed; this is just a truth about how humans are wired. Think about the last time you were upset and imagine trying to study or focus. The idea of discussing Socrates's theory of Virtue for a philosophy class and how it relates to their situation is basically impossible when you are flooded with emo-tions. So to help your friend think things through, first they need to be emotionally regulated. Maybe offer to go on a walk with them to talk, because getting outside and moving is one powerful way to help them calm down, or put on some music, grab a bite to eat, or something else that can help settle and regulate the nervous system.

4. Unless it's absolutely necessary, don't take charge of your friend's situ-ation. Ideally your friend comes up with solutions for the situation that they are going through when you create space. Allowing them to figure it out has two benefits: The first is that you don't get caught in a cycle of solving all of your friend's problems, and the second is that they are empowered when they realize they can solve most of their problems, and discover they have more strength than they'd realized. Of course, if they ask you for ideas and your help, you can offer some, but your role should be as a supporter and sounding board rather than the solver.

5. Don't just vent or "trauma bond" together. Or if you are going to vent, set a timer for two minutes to get the frustration out. Research shows that venting together makes things worse for both people. This is known as co-rumination and then begins to color the world as much darker than it is as our emotions are actually quite contagious. If you notice that your friend is venting and that you are getting caught up in it, point it out and then distract yourself with exercise or some other activity and then commit to focusing on solutions rather than venting.

6. Don't make it about you—unless they ask. Some of us, usually with good intentions, start in on telling a story about our own lives that relates to the situation. In the heat of emotion, that can be more alienating than comforting. If they are really upset, ask if they want you to share your own experiences.

Where Can We Get More Support?

There are plenty of ways to support friends, too. Sometimes it helps to activate a support network for them when you have their consent. As I'm sure you heard during orientation, there are many resources on and off campus. Maybe there's a listening service where you can get support as a concerned friend, or maybe you want to consult with your RA about what to do, or even reach out to the counseling center to ask for some help in supporting this friend. Often teammates tip off coaches about a teammate they have concerns about, or they speak to an advisor or professor they are close to. You may also check in with other friends in the group or roommates about their thoughts, and in that way you can often get a better picture of what's happening and some ways to support this person. While you may not know the parents or the relationship your friend has with their parents, many students have reported to us success when they've reached out to siblings or old high school friends of the person they are worried about to enlist them for help and support. There are many ways to not be alone with your concerns.

> I was really worried about my big's cutting, disordered eating, and other behavior, but didn't know where to look for help. With some other sisters, we actually reached out to her sibling and a high school friend of hers, and were able to get some more background on her past struggles. Since we were newer friends, her old friend actually ended up confronting her more directly with the help of her sister and she was able to get back into counseling.
>
> **—Deirdre, sophomore at a large Christian southern university**

Of course, if you are really concerned about your friend's safety, you always want to go to a professional, not just check in with other peers and friends.

Can I Actually Help a Friend Get Help or Make a Change?

In the end, no one can get help or make a change unless they themselves are motivated. Regardless of whether it's academic, social, or mental health struggles, convincing a friend to get help and make changes can be incredibly difficult. You might have encountered the "stages of change"[1] theory in one of your psychology classes, or "motivational interviewing," and these can be helpful here to think about how to support someone.

Remember, your job is not to fix them or force them into therapy, but maybe part of your role can be warming them up to the idea of getting help, and someone else can get them there. Either way, you're helping. What's great about the "stages of change"[2] theory is that it doesn't have to be about getting through all the stages at once, just nudging them one stage at a time toward the next one.

Let's imagine you are encouraging someone to seek therapy for a struggle they are having with anxiety. It's also not about guilt trips or shame. Helping someone through stages of change is about offering loving care and support, using "I statements," listening, and validating their experience along the way, not about "tough love" to push them into change.

What Are the Stages of Change?

Precontemplation. This is when the person does not even recognize the problem they are facing. When they are in this stage, you want to just help them learn a bit about the problem. They may not even know that loss of appetite or trouble with focus could be anxiety symptoms. You might educate them or share your thoughts about benefits of therapy as you've seen it help others or even yourself. In this way you can help them move toward . . .

Contemplation. People in this stage are starting to think about making the change or starting therapy or medication for their anxiety. You might point out how their mental health has changed, or how they've done hard things in the past. They are seeing more pros than cons to getting help, and they are aware that their issue is impacting friendships and academics. Discussing pros and cons of getting help may be helpful to nudge them toward . . .

Preparation. The person is now really wanting to make a change, but maybe not sure how. You can offer to go to a teacher's assistant (TA) session with them and point out resources you know have helped others (or even yourself). You might ask how you can help, offer to help them set up an appointment, or walk them over after class when they can begin to take . . .

Action. This is when the person actually begins to make the change, like starting therapy. Here you can continue to help them remember appointments or medication, help with the finances or insurance logistics if you are a caregiver, and remind them that you are proud of the work they are doing and changes they are making to their life. Again, they are the ones that need to take the action, but you can be there to make that easier for them until they are able to be more in . . .

Maintenance. Hopefully the person is continuing to progress and not backslide into their red flags or old struggles. As a supportive person, you can remind them of the positive changes they've made, the coping skills they've picked up along the way, and anticipate challenges and making coping plans for the anxiety that comes with finals, or other people, places, and things that trigger their anxiety. Give specific complements and feedback on what they've done well to care for themselves and the strengths you admire about them.

Termination. At this phase, the active work might wind down with positive changes made. You can celebrate with the person the progress they've made and continue to discuss their coping skills. Some models also discuss *relapse*, as many folks might struggle with the ups and downs of an ever-changing life that impacts their mental health as well, and it's important as a support person to not blame your friend or child, but help them back on track to the stage of change where they are getting the fullest support they need.

How Else Can I Learn to Be a Better Listener or Support?

If you want more experience helping others, campuses and the communities around them often have volunteer opportunities where you can learn some basic first aid and psychological first aid. Many campuses have EMT trainings, for example, where you can get firsthand experience for a range of emergencies. You might also sign up to be an RA, a peer leader, or a peer counselor, which also often come with some counseling training. Psychological first aid classes are also often offered. Campuses and local communities also often have emergency hotlines for people who are struggling with a range of issues, and there are many national crisis hotlines and text-lines as well. You might also want to work or volunteer at a group home, mental health facility, or homeless shelter. Many churches, temples, and spiritual communities have some informal counseling and outreach opportunities as well. You could also consider mentoring or tutoring local students who may need an older mentor to listen just as much as they need academic support. And, of course, on a campus of a research university, there may be opportunities to research mental health and work directly with research participants on new treatments. Any of these will build your empathy, counseling, and listening skills in ways that can help you be a better friend and support to others.

A Word About Fentanyl and Drug Overdoses

Let's be real: You are likely to find almost any drug on your campus, but we want to single out the drug fentanyl for reasons that will become clear if you aren't already familiar. Fentanyl is a synthetic opioid that is 50 to 100 times more potent than heroin or morphine.

In the United States, fentanyl is a leading cause of death in young people. Nearly 200 people are dying from fentanyl overdoses every single day. According to the Centers for Disease Control and Prevention, fentanyl was involved in the overwhelming majority of youth overdose deaths in 2021, and this crisis has followed teens onto college campuses. The reason that fentanyl is so dangerous is that it not only stops a person from breathing, but it also overrides the signal to breathe when carbon dioxide levels get too high, leading to suffocation.

Most students don't even take fentanyl intentionally, but many drugs (even prescription drugs) received illegally come from counterfeiters who increase profits by making pills or selling drugs made of or cut with fentanyl. So, while students may think they're taking pure substances like opiates, benzodiazepines, or MDMA, some are laced with or made with fentanyl.

The first thing is that you need to know what you're using or experimenting with, and given the statistics, you have to assume that any pill that has not been directly purchased from a pharmacy could contain fentanyl. Even if someone tells you that what they're giving you is safe because it is a prescription drug or because they've tried some themselves, it is better to assume that it is laced. Remember that the drug producers' intention is to profit from your addiction, and yet the smallest amount of fentanyl could kill you.

But there is good news. For one, you can get test kits for your recreational drugs that are available online, in the pharmacy, or in local health centers. For another, there are drugs that can rapidly reverse the effects of fentanyl (or other opiates) known as naloxone, or more commonly as Narcan, that are also available in the aforementioned locations. Naloxone is an FDA-approved medication that can be used to temporarily reverse opioid overdoses. It is administered through a nasal spray or as an injection. Although it does reverse the effects of fentanyl and helps the person start breathing again, the benefit is only temporary and can wear off quickly, so additional doses might be necessary. If a friend stops breathing or appears to be overdosing, you should call 911 immediately. Follow the instructions on the naloxone packaging and the training you received and wait for help.

Many college campuses have recognized that the fentanyl epidemic is impacting their students and have made drug test kits and naloxone freely available on campuses. If you or your friends are engaging in recreational drug use, we strongly encourage you to inquire with your college health center about how to get drug test kits or naloxone, or seek them out yourself. Try to have more than one drug test kit and dose of naloxone on hand just in case. In college, experimentation is often a part of the experience, so if you or your friends are going to engage, do your part to make that engagement as safe and intentional as possible.

In Conclusion

When we care about someone, we may want to solve it all, offer immediate solutions and advice, or share from our experience. But you can also slow down, ask your friend if they want one of the "Three H's" in a challenging moment—to be hugged, helped, or heard. And then respect that!

You can draw from your experience, experiences of others, and from the previous "maintaining your gains" chapter for ideas as well. But oftentimes, the best approach is to listen, validate, and simply just be there with them in their experience. And if you're uncertain, simply ask, "Do you want someone to listen right now, or do you want some advice or help?" Remember, stages of change remind us that we don't have to solve everything at once, and most importantly, we also need to remember to take good care of ourselves when we're caring for others, too.

Chapter 8
Feeling Different, Being Different

We have included this chapter on difference because the world that we live in presents more challenges for students who are *not* white, *not* a man, *not* heterosexual/straight, *not* cis-gendered, *not* wealthy, *not* native English speakers, *not* American, *not* in perfect health physically or mentally, and maybe what we call *neurodivergent* with a brain that works a bit differently from many peers. We cannot be separated from the sociopolitical context in which we live. It can feel isolating or even impossible at times to make it through the day navigating all of the structures in American society that have been erected by those whose life experiences do not match your own. Sure, depression might be universal in some regards, but it often shows up differently for those in marginalized groups and needs to be treated differently, too. We all might experience some anxiety in social situations, but there is a distinct anxiety living within those whose lives society deems to be lacking in value because they are the "wrong" color, don't act in a "normal" way, or are attracted to the "wrong" people. All things "college," no matter how many signs and stickers there are on campus declaring how open and supportive people are, are not immune to these injustices.[1,2,3,4,5,6]

What if you want to join the support group nearby, but you're in a chair and it's on the second floor of a building that is not accessible? How do you motivate yourself to apply for internships when many are unpaid or low paid, while your friends' parents cover their rent? How could you feel like you fit in when what you want to fit into is different from many of the other students?

It's exhausting to be different. But it can be gratifying to feel connected to who you truly are. When we accept and settle in with who we are, it can feel like life is somehow opening up for us, and we feel liberated. And it's never been easier to find community around identity. Thanks to social media, in an instant, we can find people like us, and many campuses are more likely than ever to have various affinity groups and resources for those in need. But as these differences become magnified, it might also feel even more disheartening and frustrating to belong to a marginalized group. It might raise questions for you, such as "Why do I have to work extra hard to stay on top of my mental health?" or "Why does no one care that I have to experience the world this way?" and "Why can't I get professional help from people with similar lived experiences?" On the one hand, greater visibility of these issues can make you feel supported and resilient; on the other hand, it can be demoralizing to know that this is a reality that you have to face everyday. And finally, even within these groups, how often are people seen as having the same experience when that's not always the case? Kojo, a junior from Ghana, shared,

> I grew up in a traditional conservative home in Ghana. When I became depressed, my family prayed to my ancestors to help me, and I had never heard of talk therapy back home. My therapist at college told me to join an organization to be more connected. She recommended that I join a Black student campus organization, but I found that I had more in common with foreign students from Africa than I did with the Americans. We are not all the same.

This chapter won't solve all of these issues. But our hope (as either members of these groups or allies) is that you can feel seen and validated, and that this chapter and the voices within can help you navigate the unique challenges for your mental health. We hope it can connect you to any parts of your identity that might require extra care, and that it inspires you to find community with those who can understand your experiences so you can access a sense of connection and belonging. Whether it is through a formal support group, informal support through peers, social media, or even just reading a book by and for those in your group on your own, we believe feeling understood and seen, and experiencing a sense of connection and belonging, will go a long way in supporting your efforts toward wellness.[7,8,9]

How Do I Manage Mental Health *and* My Marginalized Status?

When you belong to one or multiple marginalized groups, the college experience can become more harrowing than it already is with all of its demands and

"Welcome to Adulthood" experiences. If you're reading this book, chances are that you already belong to at least one marginalized group because you're dealing with mental health. But many of us live at the intersection of more than one identity, and this adds challenges. This is called intersectionality. Collins and Bilge define it as follows: "Intersectionality investigates how intersecting power relations influence social relations across diverse societies as well as individual experiences in everyday life.... [It] views categories of race, class, gender, sexuality, nation, ability, ethnicity, and age—among others—as interrelated and mutually shaping one another."[10]

If we apply this to the college experience, we can say that there will be some shared realities between two students who are on the autism spectrum. But if one is a white cis-gendered man who comes from a low-income family with parents who did not attend college, and the other is a Latina trans woman who comes from an upper-middle-class family with parents who did attend college, it's possible they both might need some of the same things to make college work for them, but given that they have other identity factors that differ, they will also require some things that aren't the same. You might notice that this holds true for you, too.

In this chapter, we hope that you will consider how different identities impact your experience at college as you also try to tend to your mental health. We share some general advice for all students belonging to marginalized groups, but we've also shared some specific information for specific groups.

General Guidance for Students in Marginalized Groups

- **Prioritize your well-being.** College requires an outpouring of energy and effort that can feel never-ending right up until a semester's end. While it might seem obvious, it can be easy to forget to add in a sprinkle of self-care while you make your way through. If it's dancing (which was recently found to be particularly effective for relieving depression),[11] journaling about your feelings at the start or end or your day, or even just taking three deep breaths before you leave your room, try to commit to doing something nourishing for yourself every day. Even just the smallest, simplest thing can help!
- **Locate and use your resources.** Sometimes those who need them the most use them the least. Does that sound like you? You'll never know if there is a way to make life easier if you don't reach out or try what's available to you with your tuition. Often it's easy to identify the problem, but what about taking that first step toward a solution? Who can you call

or email for help before your first class tomorrow? Which office can you stop by after class tomorrow for support? We challenge you to take that first step.

Do you not even know where to start? Ask your advisor or dean to point you in the right direction or ask a mental health professional if they have any ideas, or even classmates or resident advisors (RAs). Asking around is the first step toward finding out what's available to you. This is also great practice for "the real world" you hear about coming after graduation.

- **Find a mentor.** A mentor can lead to a lot of positive outcomes: better relationships, improved career possibilities, higher self-esteem, and higher levels of motivation.[12] For those in marginalized groups, it can be especially impactful. Some colleges offer mentoring programs for marginalized groups with older students and graduates. But even if your college doesn't have a program, there are other options—the big in your fraternity or sorority, the team captain, the RA. Is there a professor whom you look up to, or some other staff member at school? Visit their office hours or reach out to see if you can connect with them more. Or is there a field that you'd like to enter, but you don't know anyone in it? See if there is someone in the alumni network at your college that you can connect with through a directory or your college's career center. Attend that talk with the person visiting your college who does your dream job and go up to them afterward. They wouldn't be on campus if they didn't expect to meet students and have them reach out later. Do some searching on LinkedIn and send a message to anyone who seems interesting. Find a company or organization that sparks your interest. Or even just spend time with an older student whom you admire and see if they can provide you with any guidance. If all of that seems like too much, or you don't find someone through any of those avenues, even just reading a book or watching content with inspiring people can help keep you going. Chelsie and Chris met in an alumni Facebook group when she reached out for mentorships, and now we're coauthors!

- **Find or build community and belonging.** There's nothing like having people around you who get it. For students in marginalized groups, experiencing a sense of belonging in college can bring about higher academic achievement, persistence, and better mental health and self-confidence.[13,14] Have you looked into the affinity or cultural groups or affinity housing? Sometimes those groups can feel cliquey, or themselves have their blind spots about intersectionality, so shop around. If there aren't any that feel right, could you create one yourself or petition for it? If it feels overwhelming, see if a friend is open to sharing the weight of trying to make your idea happen. Does your college's counseling center have support groups for students sharing your identity, or is there an office (perhaps a Diversity, Equity, Inclusion, and Belonging [DEIB] office) or some sort of center that offers programming geared toward students like you? Ideally, your college will already have programs, organizations, or other resources that are meant to support students like you, but sometimes you might have to take the initiative to create and foster those spaces and opportunities.

- **Engage in advocacy.** When you're feeling helpless, try helping yourself and others. If you think that you would benefit from specific support that you are unable to receive, are experiencing discrimination, or have witnessed some other injustice, make moves toward the outcome you're wanting. Just because something doesn't exist or isn't happening right now, doesn't mean that it can't or won't! If we stop dreaming of and pushing for better realities, we'll never have them (you can find more on this in Chapter 6.)

What Advice Have Students Shared About Being Black, Indigenous, and People of Color (BIPOC)?

- **What do you love about being [insert your racial identity here]?** At times when you might be feeling down (because dealing with overt and covert racism definitely take their toll), it's important to remember the reasons why you may love aspects of your family, culture, or identity. Is it your people's music? Dancing? Food? Humor? Wisdom? Something else? Remember those things when you feel like you don't belong because, guess what? What you do belong to is a lineage of beauty and resilience.
- **It's okay to be frustrated with racism and racist societal structures.** It can be exhausting to exist in a world where you must, or feel called to, code switch, translate yourself, pretend to be someone you're not, educate those who are ignorant, advocate for yourself or your people, or wonder if you're behaving in a certain way that will reinforce a stereotype, and much more. You're subject to certain painful experiences that folks in the dominant group don't have to face, and you're allowed to feel your real feelings about this. There is an ease with which white people can generally move through North American institutions that were built

for them,[15] and this naturally can lead to some frustration. Rely on community for shared understanding. You don't need to add any pressure to yourself to be "okay" with it.

Sometimes it doesn't even feel like real life here because it is so different from home and the other students don't get a lot of things from my perspective. It's like I live in a different world and speak a different language. Code switching is exhausting. When I go back home or I'm with my other Black friends, it feels like I'm turning off the Brittany I have to be in most of the environments at school. But it also has made me appreciate my family and friends even more because I can be myself around them.

—Brittany, first-year student at a medium-sized private university

What Advice Have International Students Offered?

- **Bring home to your new home.** Whether it is bringing your favorite objects from home, hanging up a poster or picture of where you're from, or indulging in meals from your culture, try to surround yourself with reminders of home for each of your five senses. Watch your favorite TV show. Listen to the music. Share your culture with other students by cooking your favorite meal from home for your roommate, start a new affinity group, or plan a cultural event. Find your cuisine locally or discover a cultural/religious organization that relates to your culture— you'll likely find others from your community gathering there, students and nonstudents alike.
- **Stay connected to family and friends.** It is difficult to find time for anything while you're in college, let alone making plans to talk to someone who might be in a very different time zone! Whether it is through text, a phone call, a video chat, social media, or video games, try to set aside the time. As soon as you get your class schedule, identify time periods that overlap with ideal times to communicate with folks from home. See if you can schedule them in regularly to keep the connection alive. Maybe they can call or video call you from somewhere in your town or city so you can hear or see those familiar aspects of home.

It was hard to make friends with the American students, and it felt like the American students would stick together. I started to offer tutoring to students in my language. It helped me meet students and feel more confident to branch out. I even started a movie series in my dorm to showcase Japanese films. I ended up making friends with some of the students who I encountered, which also helped introduce me to other students.

—Misaki, junior at a small liberal arts college

How About Dealing With Being Low Income as a Student?

- **Fear of missing out (FOMO) is real.** If you don't have the means to buy the new thing, order takeout, travel over breaks, or do unpaid or low-wage internships to get ahead, it sucks. There is no getting around that. Cry, ugly cry, angrily write in your journal, vent to your friends who also can't afford these things, or don't have those opportunities or connections. Get it out, and only *then* focus on three things that you're grateful you do have. Still feeling some resistance? Let yourself feel those other feelings a bit more first. But once you've exhausted them, write out three things that you're grateful to have. Is it free (kind of free, anyway) food at the dining hall that's pretty good and available when you need it? Your own room? Something else? Reflect on those three things that you're enjoying about this weird new world. And remember gratitude is not pretending things are good or fair when they're not—it's acknowledging the suck of all of it, but taking in the good where we can find it.
- **Get creative about ways to meet your needs.** When you know that something is either not an option or might be difficult to attain, ask yourself this question: What do I *really* need? Let's pretend that you say, "To go on the trip to Mexico for spring break." Why do you want to go? Is it to spend time with your friends? To experience a new place? To eat the food? Whatever your reason is, there is a deeper need underneath. If you want to go to spend time with your friends, perhaps you have a need for belonging or connection or laughs. Maybe you're craving adventure and new experiences. For the food, besides needing to satiate your hunger, it could be a need for excitement. With all of these underlying needs (belonging, connection, humor, adventure, stimulation, excitement), aren't there many other ways to experience them? You could also experience a sense of belonging, connection, and humor by spending time with your other friend who can't afford to go, or video chatting with your friends from home if you're stuck on campus over the break. You could try meeting your needs for adventure, stimulation, and excitement by taking a walk to a neighborhood or nearby spot you never go to or by taking a bus ride into the city. Even a new book or video game might do it. It still sucks (we're not encouraging

you to pretend that it's all fine), but hopefully if you pause to try to find the underlying need and get creative about ways that you can meet it, it'll get you through these disappointing moments.

Growing up, I rarely had my own space. Sometimes that meant sleeping on the floor in the living room, sharing a room with my mom and sister at one of my mom's friends' homes, or even sleeping in the car. When I went to college, I felt so lucky! For the first two years I had a two-room double, so I basically had my own room. And then for the second two years, I had my own room. Even though most of my friends could afford to buy or do things that I couldn't, which meant that I felt left out or upset at times, I was always so happy to have my space to myself.

—Chelsie, coauthor

What Are Challenges and Advice for First-Generation Students?

- **No question is a dumb question.** Yes, we've all heard this at some point, but you need to hear this because not having caregivers (or maybe even siblings) who have been to college can create gaps in your understanding. There might be times when it seems like your classmates have it all together and you have no idea what's going on. Or maybe they don't know what to do, but they call their caregiver who went to college, get some guidance, and keep going. There will be times when you feel uncertain about which choice to make, and we encourage you to ask away. Ask your advisor, ask your professor, ask your teaching assistant, ask your dean—ask anyone whom you need to ask to try to find your answer, or to be redirected to someone who is better equipped to answer your question. There is no shame in you not knowing how it all works, because this is all entirely new!
- **Be aware of any extra pressure to succeed.** You've made it to college, which is an incredible accomplishment. So now what? Slow down. Appreciate how amazing it is that you made it, even though your caregivers (even your ancestors) never did. Many first-generation students feel an extra pressure to do well at college, or to pursue certain majors, and, at times, that might make you feel more anxious, overwhelmed, deflated, or frustrated. Whenever you feel unhappy with your academic performance, reflect on all that you've already achieved with gratitude and pride. You have already succeeded in a lot of ways and made your

ancestors proud! First, bask in all that you've accomplished and *then* reflect on what to do different next time.

My parents were so proud of me for going to college, and I didn't want to let them down. My first year was rough. My grades were terrible, and I didn't know what I was doing. I was so overwhelmed. I felt like I couldn't breathe and had bad anxiety. I saw a therapist at my college, and she helped me realize that I was putting more pressure on myself to get a 4.0 than my parents were. I felt the weight of generations, but she helped me connect with the joy of them. She also helped me realize that I needed more help because my parents didn't go to college, so I worked on getting connected to good resources at school. After that, I got better grades, but I was also easier on myself and tried to be more positive.

—Hector, sophomore at a small liberal arts college

How Can I Cope With Confusion or Even Confidence Around Gender and Sexuality?

- **Engage in self-discovery.** If you're questioning, take your time to explore. When did you first wonder about gender? When did you first wonder about sexuality? Is there a reason why you feel confused about this? Reflect with friends, mentors, or therapists or write down your thoughts in a journal. You could also read and watch some positive stories about these topics. How does this feel to you? Liberating? Scary? Interesting? Sexy? When you're alone, how does it feel to enact this part of yourself? Do you feel more like you're being yourself when you dress and speak this way? Does it feel awkward? Get curious about what's happening and process it on your own or with others (i.e., therapist, friend, support group, online community), up to your comfort level. There's no need to rush to figure it all out—let the answers come to you, and let them change as you change.
- **Explore and experiment.** Once you feel safer exploring this on your own, then you can test it out. Experiment with leaving your room in the clothes that you prefer, or by sharing your crush with a trusted friend. It's okay if you aren't ready to be loud about it yet, or ever. The process is different for everyone, and you are already being brave in confronting what's happening within you, even though the thought of judgment from others (or even your own self-judgment) is arising. As you take small steps toward expressing yourself fully, you can build a greater sense of safety and confidence to keep going and take bigger

leaps. Check in with yourself along the way to see if it feels right, like you're being more you. Are you already feeling clear on your gender identity or sexuality and expressing yourself accordingly? Celebrate that! Not everyone has the courage that you do to be who they are in a world that can be disapproving and even dangerous for those who do. As you connect with community, learn more about mental health resources or particulars within the community—like the role of hormones, or any concerns you might have about confidentiality with non–mental health professionals.

I was uncomfortable with my sexuality in high school because I had grown up with all of those people my whole life, and I didn't know how my parents would react, so I pretended to be straight. Once I started college, I knew that I wanted to let myself be free, but it was an awkward transition because I never tried anything with another girl before. I made some queer friends by going to events for queer students, and I felt so seen. Having a strong queer community is so great at my college because it feels like everyone is welcome and can be authentic. It helped me be more confident.

—Chloe, senior at a large public university

Are There Ways to Manage Physical Disabilities?

- **Allow yourself to grieve.** Whether you were born this way or became physically disabled at some point in your life, getting to that "acceptance" that people talk about can feel glib or incredibly hard, especially in a world that was not built for your needs. Why are you different? Why did you choose to ride your bike that day? What if you hadn't? It can all feel so unfair, especially when you see others who don't have to struggle in the way that you do, or you remember how life was before whatever happened. Making the transition to college isn't easy when you have to think about how to navigate it with your disability. How will it impact navigating campus? Classes? A social life? Will other students treat you differently? So many worries might arise, even heavier feelings like disappointment or frustration. Let yourself feel what you need to feel about it, and use your supportive practices and networks to move through it at your own pace. Be sure to get in touch with accommodations ASAP, and consider joining activist groups to advocate for better accessibility if issues arise.

It's so annoying sometimes after my accident. Like, why do I have to deal with this brace from now until, forever or some new surgery comes along? I definitely get angry at what I can't do anymore. But my therapist helped me focus on where I don't have pain, don't have limitations, and I feel more optimistic, I take it as a challenge to love myself more. Like, nope, this is not going to ruin my life or take away everything else that I have going for me!

—Fatima, senior at a large public university

How Do Religious Students Cope in This Environment?

- **Experience your faith wherever you are.** Many colleges have staff onsite who can provide religious and spiritual guidance, called chaplains. Often, students can schedule a time to meet with them or just drop in. Not all colleges have a chaplain to support every faith, but even if that's the case, there is typically at least one chaplain who can support other faiths. Get to know them! When you're feeling in need of inspiration, they could be a great resource to keep you connected to your faith. You can always attend services on campus (if there are any), in the local community, or stay in touch with others online.
- **Commit to your practices, celebrate your holidays.** It can be difficult to find the time to make sure that you are keeping up with your religious or spiritual practices, or observing holidays. Even if it's the slightest, find your time. If it's a prayer before sleep, reading one page of a book in the morning when you first wake up, or requesting time away from your class, job, or internship, see what you can commit to and follow through. And, please avoid judging yourself if you're not the perfect [insert religious identity here]! You're doing what you can, and that matters. A spiritual study group on campus can also be empowering and bring some peace as well.

I downloaded this app that shares a verse of the day. I don't have lots of time to read for pleasure or spiritual study when classes are happening, but it's nice to have a verse to reflect on each day that conveniently pops up on my phone so I don't have to think about it.

—Asha, first-year student at a large public university

In Conclusion

Mental health is hard, and our backgrounds can be a source of strength but also a source of added stress and stigma. But the more we get to know ourselves, the more they can become the former, not the latter. The truth is that discrimination, microaggressions, and macroaggressions, intended or not, are real, they really hurt, and they can really hold us back. Finding or building support will be a unique process for you, and in your journey, who knows? You could even become a trailblazer and make the world of mental health recovery more accessible to future generations by your taking action for yourself today.

PART II

DIAGNOSIS

How Do I Use the Diagnosis Section?

We've organized these last few chapters in a way we feel is most helpful. We've got the most common diagnoses and issues students struggle with. We describe the symptoms from the *Diagnostic and Statistical Manual of Mental Disorders* (*DSM*), basically a giant book describing all mental health issues, and then provide descriptions from students themselves (flags for you) and how they look from the outside (flags for your support network).[1] Just remember, everyone experiences these symptoms to some degree; the question is how long they've been around and how much they interfere with your schoolwork, friendships, and other important things in your life. As Freud said, it's about how well you function in work and in love. So this information is provided not so that you can diagnose yourself or your friends or family, but to give you a rough sense of what to look out for. If this list resonates with your experience or what you're seeing in others, talk to an actual licensed professional or encourage the person that you have in mind to do so. *Please.*

Also remember that when you're feeling bad, there are many reasons why you might feel the way you do. One student thought she was depressed, but then changed her birth control and suddenly her depression lifted. Other students found that they had more serious medical problems like thyroid issues, and a talk with their doctor clarified the situation. And let's face it: Homesickness is very real, too, not to mention that forgetting to sleep and eat can make your emotions swing wildly as well. So don't forget to do your due diligence as you sort out what is contributing to whatever you're experiencing emotionally!

Some Words on Self-Diagnosis, Social Media, and Your Psych 101 Textbook

If you've taken an introductory psychology course, you might have learned about different biases, including one known as "The Barnum Effect." It often sticks with one even decades after barely passing Psychology 101. (We averaged a C– in Psychology 101 . . . Maybe you don't want this book?)

The Barnum Effect is when students read about a disease or illness and they begin to see the signs and symptoms in themselves, or they start diagnosing any-one and everyone around them. We include this as a reminder that, as we start looking more closely at diagnoses, you might feel tempted to diagnose yourself or other folks around you, but we encourage you to hold off. When you see a lot of these symptoms as they're described for more than a few weeks, you really ought to check in with a professional who can better and more objectively assess what's been going on. That said, you don't want to minimize any of these either.

All of us are grateful that the stigma around mental health is on the decline. And not just in North America, but as Blaise and Chris travel around the world, young people everywhere are talking openly about struggles with depression, anxiety, posttraumatic stress disorder (PTSD), and more. In fact, it's often young folks who are educating older generations about the importance of mental health, and on understandings of mental illness. A lot of this is due to an issue that we hear makes mental health worse, and that's social media.

So, yes, like almost anything else, social media can be helpful and unhelpful. It's done wonders to destigmatize mental health, at the same time as exacerbat-ing mental health and loneliness. It's helped people connect and get support, but it's also unfortunately spread tons of bad information about symptoms, self-diagnosis, and most problematically, how to best manage mental health issues. You may feel like many people in your life are minimizing your mental health struggles, but we've often seen social media maximize small symptoms as indi-cating a more severe issue, which may end up getting you the wrong treatment that can make things worse. This book and chapter is a starting, not an ending point, and a resource, not a treatment. And we've also noticed that diagnoses, accurate and otherwise, come in waves. At the time of writing this, a flurry of self-diagnosis on social media about neurodivergence was fading, while a trend of depersonalization disorder (you probably don't have it) was rising, and surely there will be another one by the time this is published.

That said, it's important to remember, too, that you might also meet the criteria for more than one diagnosis. Fortunately, a lot of therapies and even medications can be helpful for a number of diagnoses. So if you feel like there's more going on than just one diagnosis can speak to, there just might be.

We've noticed the formula that a number of social media mental health influ-encers (and other pharmaceutical companies) use to gain their followers by offering vague symptoms that almost anyone would identity with that they say match up with a diagnosis that you need to follow them or buy their product or program to get better. Often you'll find sentiments like "If you're ever nervous at a party, you could have social anxiety" or "If you ever struggle to focus, or pro-crastinate, you could have ADHD." Remember, almost everyone gets nervous at parties, and almost everyone procrastinates and struggles to focus (and these are particularly true for college students!). Make a mental note, but please check with a mental health professional before you jump to self-diagnose based off of vague criteria.

You may want to join social media support groups and communities for answers and support, too. And while we strongly encourage you to do this, make sure it's a healthy group with people who are sharing good information, stories of hope, and who are getting better.

Remember, many people who post the most and the loudest are often strug-gling the most, and they may not always be the most helpful sources of informa-tion. Folks who are improving probably use the group less frequently, so you'll find an inherent bias in the kinds of people who are most active. Consider what you are looking for in a group or community—support, resources, connections, or what. Find a balance between the group and information from professionals. Some folks in groups online and off can be very needy, and they sometimes feel threatened when others improve and find ways to hold you back from getting better. So just remember, not everyone's motives are pure, whether they realize it or not, and not everyone is getting better in online groups. Seek out groups where people are getting better, not just getting worse or treading water. It can be validating to read from others who are struggling and sometimes necessary so that we know we're not alone with what we're facing. But balance is needed!

> When I first got my diagnosis I went wayyyy too deep into social media and groups, and at first it was helpful, but then it began to feel like an echo chamber. I heard someone say, stick with groups that are in the solution not in the problem, and stick with the people who are getting better, that was really helpful in terms of not getting dragged back down again.
>
> **—Christina, college graduate with substance abuse and depression issues**

> As a parent, finding some online support groups was overwhelming at first, because so many parents are understandably so emotional. I held back a bit from sharing a lot or asking questions beyond just ones about where to find quality resources.
>
> **—Shaun, parent of a college graduate with depression**

Chapter 9

What Is Neurodivergence?

What Is Neurodivergence?

Neurodivergence is having a different brain than most of your peers, which results in perspectives and behaviors that create unique challenges socially and academically. Neurodiversity recognizes the wide variety in these differences. The conversation around neurodivergence and neurodiversity has never been more amplified than it is today, largely because of the way that attention-deficit/hyperactivity disorder (ADHD) and autism spectrum disorder (ASD) diagnoses have become more common and more understood. Why now? Perhaps this is because our society is diversifying, and norms are being questioned. Gaps in research and diagnosis rates for marginalized groups are being highlighted. Progress is being made!

But bringing your neurodivergent brain to college can feel intimidating. How will this demanding and standardized environment work for you, academically and socially? Fortunately, college environments have become more accommodating. Whether the support is technological, academic, social, or emotional, neurodiversity is being more widely recognized and accommodated, sometimes even celebrated, in higher education.[2] That doesn't mean that the adjustment will be easy—but your success is more likely now than ever before.

What Is Masking?

Some neurodivergent students have gone or continue to go undiagnosed due to "masking." Masking is when someone hides who they truly are to fit in and belong, or to appear "normal." Why would someone want to do that? It is often because of familial or societal pressures, or norms. Girls, women, and marginalized groups often feel more social pressure and might miss out on being diagnosed with ASD or ADHD because they present neurotypically, but exhaust themselves in that process. At some point, the ability to suppress or conceal their true self starts to feel impossible and begins to negatively impact personal relationships, self-care, and/or professional/educational tasks or opportunities. When this occurs, it might lead to a further investigation of one's mental health needs and, ideally, a fitting diagnosis that captures their reality.

What Is The Deal With Self-Diagnosis?

You might relate to a lot of the symptoms of ASD and wish to self-diagnose as one way to reclaim a sense of autonomy. Dealing with medical professionals can leave some feeling unheard and disregarded, especially those coming from marginalized communities, and/or those who don't fit a clean and limited description of how these diagnoses typically present, or have been researched. Many symptoms may resonate, and until you have a more formal diagnosis, you can seek out similar coping strategies as someone with a more formal diagnosis.

Sometimes it's validating to just understand yourself as neurodivergent, even without a clear label, and just that can bring a lot of relief! If you relate to the symptoms of a certain diagnosis, share them with a mental health professional. For most mental health professionals, this level of collaboration is encouraged, but bear in mind some will be skeptical of you coming in with a self-diagnosis. Regardless, exploring the coping strategies that you can find on your own might make a huge difference.

Resources

Books

- *Divergent Mind: Thriving in a World That Wasn't Designed for You* by Jenara Nerenberg
- *The Power of Neurodiversity: Unleashing the Advantages of Your Differently Wired Brain* by Thomas Armstrong, PhD

Honestly, I first saw a lot of TikToks about autism and they made me wonder if I might be autistic. I'm a Black girl from Colorado so I don't think the possibility occurred to anyone around me growing up. I was diagnosed with Bipolar Disorder as a teenager, and then it got changed to PTSD [posttraumatic stress disorder], but when I learned more about autism, I started to think that might be right. Self-diagnosis is a big thing in the autistic community, which I think is valid, and I know that there is a lot of discourse around professional versus self-diagnosing. . . . But because I was in my junior year of college and knew that my autistic symptoms, like sensitivity to noise and environments, mess with my ability to do well, I got a formal diagnosis from a psychologist so that I could get accommodations. It has improved things dramatically and has made me feel less like a failure or like something is wrong with me.

—Brandy, senior at a large city private university

I was shocked to realize how much masking I was doing before I learned that I'm autistic. I kind of had a crisis because I felt like I didn't know who I really was. It scared me. I had to figure out who I was all over again because everything felt off. The way I walked and dressed and talked and everything! I lost a lot of the friends that I had at the start of college and had to start over because I wasn't being myself before. It was hard, but now I feel much happier. I went from being an extrovert with lots of friends to spending most of my time by myself in my room which I know sounds weird because you would think the opposite would make things better. But I need a lot of time to recharge and like being alone and doing whatever I want to do. I have found new friends who are more like me, or who are understanding and don't take it personally.

—Rishi, sophomore at a large public university

What Is Attention-Deficit/Hyperactivity Disorder?

Attention-deficit/hyperactivity disorder (ADHD) is characterized by issues with attention, focus, and/or self-control, either due to inattentiveness, hyperactivity and/or impulsivity, or a combination of the two. This may be the person who struggles to pay attention, stares off into space, can't stop moving or talking, or has a difficult time seeing tasks through. Only in more recent years has it shifted away from a stereotype of it being a disorder that mostly affects boys, resulting in an uptick in diagnoses in girls.[3]

Nearly 6% of college students report having ADHD.[4] Having ADHD will present its challenges regardless, but in the college environment, it can rear its head in ways that are particularly frustrating. For many, it can bring difficulties in starting or completing assignments, focusing on reading or other activities, and receiving grades that one feels proud of.[5] Given the lack of structure at school and how challenging planning, focus, and organizational skills can be for those with ADHD, this can severely impact mental health. Cognitive behavioral therapy (CBT) and mindfulness-based or somatic-based therapies can be helpful therapeutic interventions. And often, stimulant medications and coaching sessions help, too.

But aren't we all struggling with our attention spans? Yes, it's true that attention difficulties appear to be more prevalent for all of us. Research shows that the average attention span went from about 2.5 minutes in 2004, to 75 seconds in 2012, to a median of 40 seconds in 2016.[6] Other research brings that number all the way down to 8 seconds.[7] Clearly, the world is suffering with some attention difficulties these days, but when these get in the way of taking care of yourself, disrupt school and relationships, or keep you from having even a moderately fulfilling life, that's when it might be more than just a result of the of the endless scroll.

What Does Predominantly Inattentive Mean?

The predominantly inattentive type shows up as challenges with focusing, managing attention, keeping things organized, and completing tasks. Check out the *DSM-5* criteria below to see if you or the person you're wondering about might be dealing with this type of ADHD. Five or more of the following symptoms have to be present for at least six months, and there can only be five or fewer symptoms of hyperactivity or impulsivity (which can be found in the following section).

- Both hyperactive and inattentive must include a few signs of hyperactivity before age 12.
- Symptoms showing up different places, including home, school, work, relationships, activities, etc.
- Symptoms are disruptive to work and relationships.
- The symptoms are not coming from another mental health issue.

Often appears to miss details or makes careless mistakes in schoolwork, at work, or with other activities.

Red Flags for You

- ☐ *Do you lose points on assignments because you missed some directions?*
- ☐ *At work, does your supervisor catch missing details?*
- ☐ *Do you miss deadlines, double book things, or put things in your calendar wrong?*

Red Flags for Others

- ☐ *Does this person often share that they messed up something at work, in lab, in class, or elsewhere because they missed a detail?*
- ☐ *If you are collaborating, do they miss pieces of the directions or miss appointments?*

Often has trouble holding attention on tasks or activities.

Red Flags for You

- ☐ *Are you easily distracted?*
- ☐ *Do you catch yourself staring off into space while trying to do something?*
- ☐ *Are you clumsy?*
- ☐ *Do you start an activity only to find yourself working on something else, or spacing out, so you often don't finish?*

Red Flags for Others

- ☐ *Do they jump around to different activities or tasks when you're together?*
- ☐ *Do they seem to randomly switch topics of conversation or work?*
- ☐ *Do they jump from task to task?*

Often does not seem to listen when spoken to directly.

Red Flags for You

- ☐ *Do you lose track of what someone is saying?*
- ☐ *At times, do you look at people and realize you are looking at them and not hearing what they're saying?*
- ☐ *If you're in class, do you notice yourself missing material and unable to sustain listening to the professor a lot more than others do?*
- ☐ *What about at a job, club, or organization?*

Red Flags for Others

- ☐ *When you are talking to this person, do they appear to space out or seem distracted?*
- ☐ *Do they need a recap on what was discussed in class or in a meeting, or ask later for the details?*

continued

Struggles to follow through on instructions, finish schoolwork, chores, or jobs (e.g., loses focus, side-tracked).

Red Flags for You

- [ ] *Do you often turn in assignments late or not turn them in altogether?*
- [ ] *Do you often skip steps to get things done or work or school assignments?*
- [ ] *Do you start cleaning or organizing something and end up distracted and doing something else?*

Red Flags for Others

- [ ] *Do they not finish what they start?*
- [ ] *Do they jump around from task to task, making very little progress?*
- [ ] *Are there times when they tell you they will complete something, but you later find out that they did not?*
- [ ] *Are they late a lot?*
- [ ] *Do they seem to have "time blindness" running late for things and not really gauging how much time something will take?*

Often has trouble organizing tasks and activities.

Red Flags for You

- [ ] *When you look at your to-do list or writing assignment, do you struggle with where to begin?*
- [ ] *Do others comment on how you did something "the hard way" instead in a more organized fashion?*
- [ ] *Do you constantly come up with new organizational systems that fall apart?*

Red Flags for Others

- [ ] *Do they struggle with planning their schedule and routine?*
- [ ] *Do they start and stop and switch working on different assignments or parts of assignments with no apparent rhyme or reason?*
- [ ] *Do they have organizational systems that seem impenetrable, illogical, or change often?*

Struggles with long-term tasks.

Red Flags for You

- [ ] Is it difficult for you to start almost any task or activity, whether it is cleaning or an assignment, especially if you know it might take more than a few minutes?
- [ ] Do you feel yourself struggling to get through completing tasks, feeling almost like you're "squirming" through them?

Red Flags for Others

- [ ] Are they a major procrastinator—like, more than the average student, in ways that chronically impact sleep, functioning. and success?

Often loses things necessary for tasks and activities.

Red Flags for You

- [ ] Do you often misplace keys, wallet, phone, ID, or other important objects?
- [ ] Do you ask others to help you keep track of your belongings?
- [ ] Are you often running late looking for things?

Red Flags for Others

- [ ] Do they lose things often, like ID, keys, wallet, phone, etc., maybe asking you for help finding them or run late because they were searching?

Easily distracted.

Red Flags for You

- [ ] Do sounds, notifications, and changes in your environment cause you to lose focus easily?
- [ ] Do you space out and not notice that time has passed?

continued

Red Flags for Others

☐ Are they constantly refocusing themselves on the tasks and activities that they set out to do?

☐ Are they always getting up and down and taking breaks while you try to study together?

Is often forgetful in daily activities.

Red Flags for You

☐ Do you have a hard time remembering what you did or said earlier?

☐ Is it difficult to remember what you are supposed to be doing, or where you're supposed to be, or what you were supposed to get while you were out?

☐ Do you wander off in the middle of doing something or forget what you were supposed to be doing, or went back to your room to get?

Red Flags for Others

☐ Does this person seem forgetful about plans or remember things they need?

What Does Predominantly Hyperactive Mean?

The hyperactive type typically shows up as restlessness, maybe excessive talking, or fidgeting. It can be accompanied by impulsivity, or self-control issues, that cause issues with patience or delaying gratification. Review the following *DSM-5* criteria to see if you or someone else might have this form of ADHD. If you or the person you have in mind have five or more of these symptoms and have had them for six months or more, with only five or fewer symptoms of inattention, then the predominantly-hyperactive type of ADHD might be present.

Often fidgets or squirms.

Red Flags for You

☐ Do you have a hard time staying still?

☐ Do you like to move your hands, feet, or body around in your seat?

☐ Do you like using fidget toys or touching objects when you are sitting?
☐ Do you sit in weird positions in your seat?

Red Flags for Others

☐ Are they constantly moving around or fidgeting?
☐ Do they seem squirmy, fidget, or get up and sit down frequently for no apparent reason?

Often leaves seat in situations when remaining seated is expected.

Red Flags for You

☐ Do you feel the urge to get up and walk around when you're supposed to be sitting?
☐ Do you take breaks during class or walk around fairly often?
☐ Has anyone, such as friends or past teachers, commented on how often you get out of your chair?

Red Flags for Others

☐ Do they get out of their chair often when you are with them?
☐ Or do they abruptly get up and move around?

Often feels restless and feels urge to move around.

Red Flags for You

☐ Does it seem impossible to stay still?
☐ Do you feel like you are getting so distracted when you sit still that it makes it more and more unbearable?
☐ When you try to not follow your urge to move, do you get antsy and uncomfortable?

Red Flags for Others

☐ Do you feel like it's rare to see this person stay still?
☐ Are they often getting up, moving in their seat, fiddling with something, or looking around for no particular reason?

continued

Often unable to take part in leisure activities quietly.

Red Flags for You

☐ *Are you often humming, singing, tapping your foot or fingers, or making some other sound while you're doing a task or activity?*

☐ *When you're supposed to do something calming or relaxing, do you feel restless?*

Red Flags for Others

☐ *Do they often make noises or sounds when they are just hanging out and relaxing?*

☐ *Do you notice them humming, talking, or singing to themselves?*

☐ *Do they talk or fidget in class or during movies?*

Is often "on the go" acting as if "driven by a motor."

Red Flags for You

☐ *Is it difficult for you to not be active somehow?*

☐ *Have others ever commented on how you "have a lot of energy?"*

Red Flags for Others

☐ *Do they seem like they have a boundless amount of energy?*

☐ *Are they always "on"?*

☐ *Do they seem like they are bouncing around when you go from place to place, picking things up, walking on curbs, and so forth?*

Often talks excessively.

Red Flags for You

☐ *Do you ever notice that you are talking much longer and more than others?*

☐ *Have you gotten that feedback?*

☐ *When you were younger, did you get in trouble in school, sports, or other activities for talking too much?*

Red Flags for Others

☐ *Are they way more of a talker than a listener?*
☐ *Do you get frustrated with how much they talk or notice that other people around seem to get annoyed with it?*
☐ *Do they not seem to "read the room" socially or miss cues about when it's time to stop talking or leave?*

Often interrupts or blurts out a thought.

Red Flags for You

☐ *Do you sometimes answer questions in class without raising your hand, or interrupt?*
☐ *Do you often get in miscommunications with people?*

Red Flags for Others

☐ *Do they seem impatient to speak?*
☐ *Do they misunderstand conversations or questions because they are incorrectly "filling in the blanks"?*
☐ *Are they hard to interrupt or converse with?*

Often has trouble waiting their turn.

Red Flags for You

☐ *Is it hard to be patient?*
☐ *Wait your turn in conversation group projects or games?*

Red Flags for Others

☐ *Do they get annoyed, or constantly talk about how long a line or wait is, or change lines or lanes in traffic?*

continued

Often interrupts or intrudes on others (e.g., butts into conversations or games).

Red Flags for You

☐ *Is it difficult to wait and not interrupt?*
☐ *Do people seem annoyed by you doing this, or do you apologize for it a lot?*

Red Flags for Others

☐ *Do you notice that they interrupt you or others when you're together?*

What Does Combined Type Mean?

For some people, they might have some (or all) or both the inattentive and the hyperactive type.

Resources

Productivity Apps

- Study Bunny
- Streaks
- Finch

Books

- *ADHD: The College Experience* by Arash Zaghi and Connie Mosher Syharat
- *Thriving With Adult ADHD: Skills to Strengthen Executive Functioning* by Phil Boissiere MFT
- *What Your ADHD Student Wants You to Know* by Sharon Saline
- *ADHD Toolkit for Women: Workbook & Guide to Overcome ADHD Challenges and Win at Life* by Sarah Davis and Linda Hill

I'm not an organized person, and that's one of my biggest flaws. It is worse because I'm in college. I use two planners, one on my computer and one in a paper planner. I write down all of my homework in the planner and how long I think it'll take me to complete it, and I schedule in breaks. I use the computer one for my class schedule.

—**Shay, sophomore at medium-sized private college**

I think it's important to find the right combination to get your work done. Like other people with ADHD, I can't just do my work anywhere. I like to work in the basement of the library because there aren't many people there, and I like to go right away in the morning because the longer I wait, the less likely it will be that I do anything. I bring my noise-canceling headphones and blast music because it helps me focus. I set a timer to take a five-minute break every thirty minutes or so, and then I get up and walk around or dance instead of scrolling. And then I keep going until class or lunch time.

—**Jamie, senior at a large research university**

Something that's really helped me is to focus on myself and not other people. I did a lot of comparisons before which would lead me to feel like I'll never amount to anything. ADHD has made my self-esteem not so good. . . . But my therapist taught me to only compare myself to myself. I try to remember to look back at my own progress. When I don't complete everything, or am running late on something, I remember how there was a time when I was barely able to do anything. I spend more time acknowledging what I am doing instead of what I'm not doing, which has made me more confident, and helped with my more negative thoughts, and has made me more productive.

—**Portia, junior at art school**

What Is Autism Spectrum Disorder?

Autism spectrum disorder (ASD) is a developmental and neurological disorder that impacts one's social interactions, communication and learning, and often behavior. Some of the major signs that one has ASD include significant challenges in communication and interpersonal interactions, narrow interests, repetitive behaviors, and sensory and environmental sensitivities which interfere with life. Still, just because you are passionate about some subjects, or feel you're awkward socially, is not a diagnosis. It's a lot more subtle than that.

Because much of the earlier research focused primarily on males and autism can show up differently in females, and children in the Black, Indigenous, and People of Color (BIPOC) community have historically been overlooked, some of those symptoms may have been missed.[8,9] Later diagnoses are becoming more common, which might provide relief to those who might not have their answers, though it can also lead to greater difficulties due to a lack of earlier intervention.[10] ASD is considered to be a spectrum because the symptoms have a very large range of severity.

Regardless of where on the spectrum one finds themselves, having ASD can contribute to major challenges at college and in life. About 35% of youth with ASD attend college.[11] The transition can be immensely stressful, and once there, navigating social situations, obstacles with meeting academic requirements and engaging in classroom environments, and even issues with sexual behaviors and encounters can be extra hard.[12] While this might seem discouraging, you can experiment with different supports, whether they are tools or therapies, to stay organized and focused and functioning at your best. Because there is so much variety in how ASD manifests, it's important to try out different possibilities to find your right fit. It doesn't mean that you have to do it on your own! Engage with your providers, academic support staff, and peer groups or communities for support in navigating the sea of options.

What Are The Symptoms Of ASD?

To have a diagnosis for autism spectrum disorder, one must meet the criteria below from the *DSM-5*. We've included some questions to ask yourself to see if you might be dealing with ASD, or if someone you know might be.

A. Ongoing difficulties[13] in all three areas of social communication and social interactions.

Deficits in social-emotional reciprocity.

Red Flags for You

- [ ] *Do you feel uncertain about how to engage in conversation?*
- [ ] *Confused about how to begin or end an interaction?*
- [ ] *Do you speak a lot and not let others respond?*

Red Flags for Others

- ☐ *Are they particularly awkward or even a bit odd in interactions?*
- ☐ *If you share something, do they not seem to acknowledge it, know how to respond, or start speaking about something else?*
- ☐ *Do they often not make space for others in conversation, like no "back and forth"?*

Deficits in nonverbal communicative behaviors used for social interaction.

Red Flags for You

- ☐ *Do you struggle with saying too much or too little?*
- ☐ *Do you feel unsure about how to orient your body in conversation?*
- ☐ *Do others misunderstand your tone of voice, facial expressions, or body language, thinking that you meant something that you didn't?*
- ☐ *Do you misunderstand others' body language and facial expressions?*

Red Flags for Others

- ☐ *Do body language, tone or volume, and facial expressions not seem to line up with content or emotions?*
- ☐ *Do you notice that they have a hard time reading nonverbal communications and cues?*
- ☐ *Do they make too little or too much eye contact?*

Difficulty making, maintaining, and understanding relationships.

Red Flags for You

- ☐ *Is it confusing the ways most people interact and communicate (i.e., friends, roommates, family, strangers, professors, or other authority figures)?*
- ☐ *Do you feel unsure about how to behave in different groups?*
- ☐ *Do you spend a lot of time by yourself or prefer to spend a lot of time by yourself, maybe going days without really seeing or talking to anyone?*
- ☐ *Do you struggle with making or keeping friends?*

continued

Red Flags for Others

- [ ] *Do they often keep to themselves and spend a lot of time alone?*
- [ ] *Do they have few friends or lose a lot of friendships?*
- [ ] *Do you find that they have a hard time figuring out how to interact with the different people in their life, whether it is professors, other students, family, or strangers?*

   B. Restricted, repetitive patterns of behavior, interests, or activities. (Diagnosis requires that a person meets at least two of four criteria.)

Repetitive motor movements or speech.

Red Flags for You

- [ ] *Do you ever repeat or echo back what you just heard someone say?*
- [ ] *Do you engage in repetitive movement, like having to pace, move your body parts in a particular way, spin around, or some other form of movement?*
- [ ] *Are there times you say a word, phrase, or sound repeatedly for no particular reason?*
- [ ] *Do you like to arrange and maybe even rearrange different objects in a meticulous way?*

Red Flags for Others

- [ ] *Do you notice that they tend to repetitively move certain parts of their body, like moving fingers or tapping feet?*
- [ ] *Do you hear them repeating back what you or others say to them, or notice them repeating certain words or phrases, over and over, sometimes from movies or shows?*
- [ ] *When you're with them, do you see them arranging objects (i.e., food on plate, materials on desk, etc.) with precision?*
- [ ] *Do they echo back parts of what you just said.*

Inflexibility in routines, difficulty with transitions, patterns of verbal or nonverbal behavior.

Red Flags for You

- [ ] *Are you extremely picky about foods, often eating the exact same thing?*

- [ ] *Go to the same places?*
- [ ] *Get agitated when your routine changes?*
- [ ] *Has anyone ever told you that you act like a robot?*
- [ ] *Is it difficult to move from one activity or task to another?*
- [ ] *Do you have a certain routine or order for how you like to accomplish things and feel "off" when you don't follow it?*

Red Flags for Others

- [ ] *Does this person seem to function almost automatically with little variation in speech patterns, body language, or routine?*
- [ ] *Do they always want to eat at the same place, or the same things?*
- [ ] *Are they so attached to their routine that it is difficult to make plans, or they get agitated?*
- [ ] *Is it very hard to pull them away from a task they're engaged in?*

Highly restricted, fixated interests that are abnormal in intensity or focus.

Red Flags for You

- [ ] *Do you have one or a few particular specific interests that are often not shared by many others?*
- [ ] *Perhaps these are interests that are so absorbing that you feel like you'd be happy to do them or learn about them forever.*

Red Flags for Others

- [ ] *Do they seem obsessed with one or a few particular interests or facts, often somewhat obscure or specific?*
- [ ] *Do they seem to spend a lot of time learning about or engaging in activities, or memorizing information related to these particular interests?*
- [ ] *Do you see them struggle with topics that fall outside of whatever that one interest is, or few interests are, and not notice others find their interests a bit strange?*

continued

Hyper- or hypo-reactivity to sensory input or unusual interest in sensory aspects of the environment.

Red Flags for You

☐ *Are you extra sensitive to your surroundings?*
☐ *Do certain configurations of lighting, smell, and/or sound cause discomfort and agitation?*
☐ *Are there particular textures present in clothing, flooring, bedding, or other objects that you have a strong aversion to?*
☐ *Have you ever been told that you have a low or high tolerance for pain?*
☐ *Do you have trouble feeling connected to or aware of your body?*
☐ *Are you easily overwhelmed?*

Red Flags for Others

☐ *Do they avoid going to certain places that are highly stimulating?*
☐ *Do they appear to struggle with focusing if there are a few different things happening at once (i.e., music in background, conversation, lots of movement in the space, etc.)?*
☐ *Are they more sensitive than others to pain?*
☐ *Maybe it seems like they are "overreacting" if they bump into something or get a small cut. Or, conversely, have you been surprised that they didn't appear more hurt in a more extreme situation?*
☐ *Do they often wear just comfortable loose-fitting clothes like sweatpants every day, even to social occasions?*

C. These symptoms usually appear when younger, but they can be concealed by "masking" until the stress of teen or college years makes it hard to keep up the facade.

D. These symptoms cannot be better explained by another diagnosis or developmental issue.

Resources

Websites

- Organization for Autism Research (researchautism.org)

Books

- *Unmasking Autism: The Power of Embracing Our Hidden Neurodiversity* by Devon Price

Helpful Tools

- Stimulation toys (i.e., fidget spinners, putty, pop fidget toys)
- Noise canceling headphones
- White noise machine
- Weighted blanket
- Visual timers
- Evernote
- Habitica

More than anything, I value a quiet space. I need a quiet space where I can recharge my social and mental batteries. A place that I can consider safe, where I can rest and gather my thoughts, and where I don't have to be social or do any masking. I need a fair bit of alone time to process things and think. That is my first priority. I needed to request my own space and somewhere quiet to live on campus.

—**Hugh, junior at small liberal arts college**

Most autistic people have difficulty with social interactions because they don't understand social interactions. Watching TV shows has helped me learn how to talk to people. I see what they talk about and copy it. I also don't force myself to be like everyone else. I'm not the type of person to go out and party every weekend. If I want to stay home, I just do what I want to do.

—**Noah, senior at a medium-sized research university**

I joined a support group for autistic people, and it helped a lot. It's nice to meet people who understand me and don't make me feel too weird. I am obsessed with some pretty niche interests and have a pretty weird sense of humor, but other people in the group get it. I still feel like a weird person, but I'm okay with that and have grown to love and accept that about myself.

—**Jade, sophomore at a small liberal arts college**

In Conclusion

Neurodiversity or neurodivergence is hard to define, since everyone's brain is unique. Still, there are some common differences that show up like ASD and ADHD that can help you feel less alone. In recent years, too, activists see neurodiversity as just that: not as pathology or a problem, just a difference. And it is a difference that can even have advantages, though there may be challenges that need some accommodating to be the best you that you can be. Hopefully you've gotten some ideas and resources that can help your unique self and brain manage your mental health and get the most out of your student experience despite any complexities that may come into play.

Chapter 10
Adjustment and Anxiety Disorders

This chapter covers adjustment and anxiety disorders, as they're the most common mental health issues that students face. We've also included trauma and stress here, since they have similar symptoms, and sometimes it can be hard to parse out what is what.

What Does an Adjustment Disorder Really Mean?

On the face of it "adjustment disorder" even sounds kind of flaky, but, believe us, it's not. In fact, it is one of the most common diagnoses out there. Fundamentally, adjustment disorder means that someone is having trouble adjusting to a big stressful situation. That could mean, well, moving to college, going through breakup, homesickness, struggling academically, grief, loss of friendship, or generally a strong and negative reaction to events that are out of proportion to a typical response.

Adjustment disorder shares symptoms with depression, anxiety, and emotional issues that impact functioning. It's a very real thing, and often the most likely thing a lot of students are suffering with. So before you jump to a bigger diagnosis of yourself or someone you care about, understand that adjustment disorder is very real, very painful, and thankfully very treatable.

Typically, it does not usually last as long as generalized anxiety, depression, or even dysthymia. Remember that in college, time itself gets really distorted, and a few days can feel like forever; when we are struggling, our brains almost literally can't remember what not feeling bad is like, and that feeling bad eventually does end.

To have a *diagnosis* of adjustment disorder, there needs to be a pretty big stress or change within three months, followed by symptoms that are out of proportion to the stress, in a way that significantly impacts relationships, schoolwork, and other aspects of functioning. Remember, there is almost always a pretty big stress within the past few months when you are in college!

And adjustment disorder is all over the *Diagnostic and Statistical Manual of Mental Disorders* (*DSM*) in terms of making a diagnosis; in fact, therapists are supposed to assume adjustment disorder rather than a more significant diagnosis.

So what exactly is adjustment disorder? According to the *DSM*, it needs to have the following:

    A. Emotional or behavioral symptoms within three months of a clear stress or change
    B. These symptoms or behaviors are clinically significant as they include
        1. Distress or reaction that is out of proportion to the stressful event or change
        2. Significant impairment in social, occupational, or other important areas of functioning

Red Flags for You

☐ *After a stressful event (like moving, breakup, major rejection, grief, illness, or starting college), are you having symptoms that are interfering with your life?*
☐ *For example, even months after a breakup, are you struggling to get to class and go out with friends?*

Red Flags for Your Support Network

☐ *After the person has gone through something stressful, are they having an emotional or behavioral response that seems way out of proportion even months afterward?*

Adjustment disorder has to be in relation to a big change like that described above, and it messes up your social or academic functioning in some way. It often has some symptoms of depression, some symptoms of anxiety, sometimes both, and sometimes a "disturbance of emotions," which means having out-of-proportion emotional reactions to things. It also may include "disturbance of conduct," which means that your behavior changes in ways that you or others might notice, like "you haven't been yourself lately." Of course, people change a lot during college, so just because your interests shift a lot, especially at the beginning of school as you discover new passions and lose interest in some things you loved in high school, this is not necessarily a red flag.

> Many folks dismiss adjustment disorder as a mild or not 'real' diagnosis or mental health issue, when in fact it is very painful and disruptive, because it often includes a grab bag of distressing symptoms from anxiety, depression, and other mental illnesses. It needs addressing, and quickly. This is particularly true because if adjustment disorder is left untreated, it can turn into a more severe mood or anxiety disorder, so is important to deal with ASAP.
>
> **—Maryam, psychologist in Pennsylvania**

We've spoken with many students with adjustment disorder who felt invalidated, or felt we were minimizing their concerns. We certainly hear that, but we believe it's important to proceed with caution around a stronger diagnosis for a number of reasons. The point is that you may not want a piece of paper or electronic record that has a more significant diagnosis than adjustment disorder. While, yes, there are confidentiality laws, and the Americans with Disabilities Act that should protect you, the fact is, you may not feel entirely comfortable with certain records. Again, ask your provider about this.

In a sense, adjustment disorder is about your reaction to change. That is, "is your reaction proportionate to the situation?"

> I was literally pissed off when I saw on my insurance forms I'd been diagnosed with adjustment disorder. I felt like a badly behaved middle schooler or something. My therapist explained why she put that down, and it just made sense to me, given the symptoms. It's also a reminder—don't be afraid to get counseling or therapy, even if something seems like homesickness or a breakup, or "not a big enough deal."
>
> **—Rupa, college graduate now in law school**

> My first-year roommate would not leave her room after the first few weeks of orientation. She just kept to herself, and talked only to her boyfriend on facetime every day. When they broke up, she really didn't have anyone to talk to and got more and more lonely and just stayed in her pajamas all day. My RA [resident advisor] who was a psych major thought she was depressed, and we helped her get to the behavioral health center, where she had a few sessions and told me it was actually "adjustment disorder," not full-blown depression. We're not really close, but I see her around campus now and she seems fine.
>
> **—Alexa, junior at a small liberal arts college**

What Are Anxiety Disorders?

Anxiety disorder is probably *the* most common mental illness, especially among college students. That's partly because we believe anxiety happens more to smart people. Why? Because you can think of 50 ways you'll fail the test, rather than just one or two. Of course, we then have many common types of anxiety: generalized anxiety disorder (GAD), with and without anxiety attacks, social anxiety, phobias, and others. We're mostly going to cover GAD, panic attacks, and just touch on social anxiety and phobias.

Anxiety hits about 32% of teens and young adults, and 20% in any given year. It appears to be increasing even more rapidly in teens and young adults. Anxiety also hits female-identified people a bit more than males.[1]

And anxiety of all kinds is truly debilitating. Often it leads students to avoid the anxiety triggers—social situations, academic challenges, and others—that can lead to feeling like your life is quickly spiraling downward. Other times it leads to extreme discomfort or overwhelming thoughts and feelings that make it impossible to enjoy your life, get to the dining hall, or focus clearly on something like an exam.

Remember, everyone gets a little anxious or worried. You're *supposed* to be nervous about meeting new people, living in a new situation, sharing a bathroom, raising your hand in class, or taking exams, but when it starts to interfere and your avoidance kicks into high gear is when you may want more substantial help. It also may start to annoy the people around you, whose constant reassurances and evidence they present to you to the contrary just don't seem to sink in.

In the next few pages you'll find the common clinical symptoms of anxiety as well as translations for what they might look like from the inside and outside.

What are the Cognitive Symptoms of Anxiety (From the *DSM-V*)?

Feeling Restless, Keyed-up

Red Flags for You

- [ ] *Do you feel like your thoughts are racing, your brain won't slow down, or you can't get your mind to stop?*
- [ ] *Are you always on edge?*
- [ ] *Do you have "catastrophic thoughts"—for example, if your friends are late, they must hate you or have gotten into an accident?*

Red Flags for Your Support Network

☐ *Do they have excess nervous energy—are they fidgety and can't sit still or get comfortable?*
☐ *Do they talk too much or too fast? (But this is a bit different than someone with attention-deficit/hyperactivity disorder [ADHD].)*
☐ *Do you hear them express out-of-proportion worries or jump to conclusions with terrible explanations for relatively normal events?*

Difficulty Concentrating or Paying Attention

Red Flags for You

☐ *Is it hard to focus on school, or even TV or video games?*
☐ *Does your mind go blank often, or do you feel like you forget everything you just learned?*
☐ *Do your thoughts feel jumbled—like you can't keep them straight or have anxious thoughts jumping in?*
☐ *Is procrastination worse?*

Red Flags for Your Support Network

☐ *Is their academic work suffering—is it barely or not getting done, and are grades falling?*
☐ *Are they unable to focus on chores or even fun things, such as conversations, shows, or video games?*
☐ *Do they seem more distracted and forgetful than usual?*

What are the Emotional Symptoms of Anxiety?

Worried, Fearful, or Scared

Red Flags for You

☐ *Do you just feel like something is wrong, or that something bad will happen to you, to others, or to the world?*

continued

Red Flags for Your Support Network

☐ Are they more clingy and tearful? Do they avoid places like classes, dining hall, social events, or other people?

Irritability or Anger

Red Flags for You

☐ Is everyone and everything more annoying, or do things get on your nerves more lately?
☐ Do you have a "short fuse?"

Red Flags for Your Support Network

☐ Are they less patient, more frustrated, and more annoyed?
☐ Are they snapping at friends, family, or roommates, or complaining about petty issues?

What are the Physiological Symptoms of Anxiety?

Easily Fatigued

Red Flags for You

☐ Are you tired more often, or do you find doing simple things exhausting?

Red Flags for Your Support Network

☐ Do they look tired, give up more easily, and have less energy for academics, socializing, exercise, and activities?

Psychomotor Agitation or Muscle Tension

Red Flags for You

☐ Does it feel like you heart is pounding really loud, hard, and fast?
☐ Are your hands sweaty (or cold and clammy)?
☐ Do you feel jittery, shaky, or have butterflies in your stomach?

Red Flags for Your Support Network

☐ *Do they seem jittery or jumpy, with hands shaking or legs bouncing?*
☐ *Is there more nervous tapping or fidgeting, or moving around and pacing?*

Somatic Distress

Red Flags for You

☐ *Does your neck (or head, jaw, and back) hurt?*
☐ *Is your stomach more upset than usual?*
☐ *Do you have more throat pain or reflux?*

Red Flags for Your Support Network

☐ *Do they complain about mysterious aches and pains, gastrointestinal distress, frequent trips to the bathroom, or frequent headaches?*

Sleep Disturbances

Red Flags for You

☐ *Do you have trouble falling or staying asleep, or waking up early?*
☐ *Do you have trouble waking up or sleep a lot but are still tired?*
☐ *Is worry keeping you up or waking you up?*

Red Flags for Your Support Network

☐ *Do they look or seem tired, or maybe jittery from exhaustion plus caffeine?*
☐ *Do they complain about sleeping?*
☐ *Do they pace or get up a lot at night?*

Appetite Changes

Red Flags for You

☐ *Do you have a nervous stomach, where the thought of eating makes you feel sick, or you are never hungry anymore?*
☐ *Or are you eating a lot more than usual to manage feelings and relax?*

continued

Red Flags for Your Support Network

☐ *Do they seem to be eating too little or too much?*
☐ *Do you notice their weight or shape fluctuating?*

What are the Treatments for Anxiety?

The most common and effective therapies for anxiety are typically cognitive behavioral therapies and mindfulness-based therapies. These might include acceptance and commitment therapy (ACT), rational emotive behavior therapy (REBT), cognitive behavioral therapy (CBT), dialectical behavioral therapy (DBT), and mindfulness-based therapies like mindfulness-based stress reduction (MBSR) or somatic experiencing (SE) (more on these in Chapter 4), and there are medications that can help, too.

The more recent therapies tend to emphasize that you *have to act your way into a new way of feeling*, rather than just try to think your way into a new way of feeling or acting. Basically, variations on exposure therapy or facing your fears will push you out of your comfort zone, but into a place that's still within your safety zone. Don't worry: No therapist should make you do things against your will, but they will encourage you to do hard and uncomfortable work, outside of your comfort zone but always within your safety zone, and they might be able to be there with you or help you find people who can help you through your fears.

Many students end up avoiding more and more of what makes them anxious because, well, why would you ever want more anxiety? It makes perfect sense. Unfortunately, this only makes your anxiety worse. You truly need to face your fears, slay your demons, lean in, walk into the eye of the storm, or whatever metaphor works for you! You just gotta do it! But we therapists are here for you.

Ahmed, a junior, was incredibly anxious about his schoolwork, which often just led to more avoidance, taking incompletes, and digging himself further into a hole. He didn't even know what grades he'd gotten for the last three semesters because he was too anxious to look, or even what assignments he was missing in the semester that we first started meeting. Over the course of our work together, we helped him feel comfortable doing some relaxation exercises before we checked his grades together. They were not great, but not as bad as he'd expected. We also composed an email to his professors to see what assignments he was missing, sat on it for a week or two, then sent it together from my office. His confidence grew, and we made a plan for getting back on top of his work, so gradually his anxiety subsided. While not strictly CBT [cognitive behavioral therapy], we were doing something like exposure and response prevention therapy, building his confidence to do those difficult things that were so hard for him while he practiced relaxation and mindfulness to not go into panic mode.

—**Chelsie, describing a client**

I think I definitely felt a pressure to succeed when I started college. It sounds one-dimensional, but it felt tied up in shame of not being good or doing well. I felt a lot of pressure. I also was comparing myself to other people—why am I going through this and not able to focus? I felt like everything that I was doing was shit. My college is rigorous, so I felt a pressure to be perfect. To have good grades, be interesting, and do well in my social life, join a lab and get research experience. . . . It just felt like I had to be perfect in everything. And with social media, you're not just confined to your own circle and you just see people working so hard and being so happy. . . . When I'm overworked, I feel like, "I can't do this anymore." Getting outside and getting exercise really helped me move out of my anxiety.

—**Niall, senior at a large research university**

What Are Panic Attacks?

Many people will have a panic attack at some point in their lives, and unfortunately, college is often when the first ones occur. Without knowing what they are, many students are overwhelmed and frightened by the physical symptoms of panic, which only exacerbate the anxiety. You might have even experienced a panic attack and not known that's what is was. Because the symptoms are so physical, many students wonder if they are having a heart attack, asthma attack, food poisoning, overdose, or something else. They certainly can be brought on by substances, and you are also more vulnerable when under the influence or withdrawing from and hungover from certain substances.

So What Exactly Is a Panic Attack?

A panic attack is a sudden surge of intense fear or discomfort that peaks within minutes and includes at least four of the following:

- Palpitations, pounding heart, chest pain (many people think they are having a heart attack)

continued

- Sweating
- Trembling or shaking
- Sensations of shortness of breath or smothering (people may worry they are having an allergic reaction)
- Feelings of choking or suffocating
- Nausea or abdominal distress (you might wonder if you have food poisoning)
- Feeling dizzy, unsteady, lightheaded, or faint
- Derealization (feelings of unreality) or depersonalization (being detached from oneself)
- Fear of losing control or "going crazy"
- Fear of dying
- Numbness or tingling sensation
- Waves of hot or cold

Red Flags for You

- ☐ *Are you sweating, shaking, or having trouble breathing?*
- ☐ *Is your heart pounding, or do you have tightness in your chest or feel sick to your stomach?*
- ☐ *Are you experiencing waves of heat or cold, waves of numbness or weird sensations, dizzy or light-headedness, or feel almost outside of your body?*
- ☐ *Do you have an overwhelming, sudden, and real feeling like you are dying, losing control, or going crazy?*

The big red flag to not worsen your anxiety is avoidance. You want to get treatment so you don't end up avoiding the situations where you worry the panic attack may happen.

Red Flags for Your Support Network

- ☐ *Is the person sweating, shaking, or having trouble breathing?*
- ☐ *Are they describing their symptoms, or asking if you think they are having a heart attack, going to die, or telling you they think they are going crazy?*
- ☐ *Do they look agitated, with a flushed or pale face?*

So these are panic attacks. They are pretty miserable, and many people will experience them occasionally, but when they happen often, the diagnosis is panic disorder.

My first panic attack was after the first time I got high in college. Where I grew up we just smoked schwag weed, and then when I went to Colorado and it was legal from the dispensary, I got waaaaaay more fucked up than I thought, and starting panicking. My heart was pounding, I felt like my throat was closing up, I couldn't breathe and was nauseous, and I thought I was having an allergic reaction to something I ate at the dining hall. I literally thought I was dying. My roommates called 911, and I was super embarrassed afterwards because it was a panic attack brought on by the weed. I actually now don't smoke anymore, because it now always makes me anxious, which kind of sucks.

—Andrew, senior at a large public university

I was at a party sophomore year and just started to feel all tunnel vision, dizzy and tingly. I wondered if someone had put something in my drink, so went home with a friend to be safe. But when it kept happening when there weren't drinks, I told my therapist and learned it was a panic attack. After that I started worrying they would happen in class, and I almost stopped going to class because I was so worried I'd throw up in front of the whole class. But with some relaxation, breathing and mindfulness stuff I learned in therapy, it's not been much of an issue since then.

—Yuri, college graduate who majored in finance

Dan called us junior year hysterically crying and saying he thought he was having a heart attack. As a nurse, I remembered from ER [emergency room] rotations that people often come in thinking they are having a heart attack because of chest pains when it's at least as often a panic attack. Nancy and I talked him down as he took a walk around campus and went to the counseling center the next day where he got some medication and CBT [cognitive behavioral therapy].

—Adam, parent of a recent liberal arts graduate

Treatment for Panic Attacks

For many people, progressive muscle relaxation and breathwork, mindfulness-based therapies, and CBT help a lot. In addition, medications like selective serotonin reuptake inhibitor (SSRIs) can help underlying anxiety, and sometimes beta blockers and benzodiazepines are recommended as needed.

What Is a Social Anxiety Disorder?

Some degree of social anxiety, sometimes called social phobia, is a given at college. Worrying about fitting in or how you are being perceived in a completely new social environment is an understandable response, and social media doesn't help! But when overwhelming anxiety comes from almost all interactions and interferes with your ability to make and enjoy social connection, a critical human need, it might be time to seek support. And while it might seem like everyone thinks they have social anxiety, the fact is that 12% of people will have to face it in their lives. It is also a little more frequent in female-identified people.[2]

Social anxiety disorder tends to show up in—you guessed it—social situations. This can be both in person, like at a party or in class, or digitally. It is also not limited to speaking with others; it can be experienced when walking through a public space, or eating, drinking, or doing other activities in a space where you can be seen. It often brings excessive thoughts about how you are being perceived in your interactions with others, leading you to avoid more and more, or feel that you must tolerate extreme feelings of fear that are disproportionate to the activity you're engaging in. There often is a worry that you will be rejected, that you will somehow offend someone, be made fun of, or end up feeling embarrassed.

The *DSM* describes social anxiety with the following symptoms:

Marked fear or anxiety about one or more social situations in which the individual is exposed to possible scrutiny by others.

Red Flags for You

- [ ] Do you having debilitating fear about meeting new people or about conversations with hallmates, classmates, and professors?
- [ ] Are you overly self-conscious about being observed—walking around campus, speaking in class, even just eating food?

Red Flags for Your Support Network

- [ ] Do they look really overwhelmed in certain situations?
- [ ] Are they excessively clingy or ask to go home from social situations?
- [ ] Are they staying in and isolating?
- [ ] Do they avoid situations where people might notice them, or frequently cover their face or hide?
- [ ] Do they seem excessively insecure or self-conscious, to the point that they avoid situations altogether, or drink/use heavily to manage?

Social situations almost always lead to significant fear or anxiety. The fear or anxiety is out of proportion to the actual threat posed by the social situation and to the sociocultural context. The social situations are avoided or endured with intense fear or anxiety.

Red Flags for You

☐ *This really means that it's not just the first few minutes of the party or class— it's the whole time, basically every party, gathering, or class. That means even the ones where you're not being evaluated by the professor or the frat or sorority members and so forth. But it's so intense that you either leave situations or avoid them altogether, even ones where you know and trust people.*

Red Flags for Your Support Network

☐ *Do they express unrealistic concerns about how they are being judged in low-stakes settings, or even by friends and classmates when they are out?*

The fear, anxiety, or avoidance causes clinically significant distress or impairment in social, occupational, or other important areas of functioning.

Red Flags for You

☐ *You are so overwhelmed with anxiety that you literally can't think. The anxiety is so bad that it damages your social standing and academic performance.*

Red Flags for Your Support Network

☐ *You're getting really concerned that this is impacting the person's social or work life. Now people are maybe avoiding them, or not bothering to invite them because they never go, act strangely, or leave events quickly. They may be not going to class either, or the gym, or even to the dining hall.*

The fear, anxiety, or avoidance is persistent, typically lasting for six months or more. This has to be ongoing, not the adjustment anxiety and social roller coaster that many students experience the first few months of school.

continued

Red Flags for You

☐ Do you constantly check who engages with your social media posts and have big feelings about it?

☐ Do you avoid social media altogether because being perceived is too much?

☐ Do you spend a lot of time in your dorm room?

☐ Do you have to have nicotine, alcohol, weed, or other substances to make social interactions bearable?

☐ Do you hold your breath while in social settings or avoid walking through your campus where you might be seen?

☐ Do you cancel plans with friends, ghost people, or avoid parties or other events?

☐ Do you get sweaty when you have to go to social engagements, or do you trip over your words when speaking?

☐ Do you start to get nervous even just thinking about speaking, walking, and/or doing other activities in front of other people?

☐ Do you avoid dating or hookups, even though you'd like to enjoy them?

Red Flags for Your Support Network

☐ Does the person often cancel plans to hang out or seem disengaged or stressed when they spend time with you?

☐ Is your friend typically more shy and reserved, but then drinks too much alcohol at social outings to become more extroverted?

☐ Do they overanalyze social situations and describe them in a much more negative light?

☐ Do they avoid speaking in class and engaging with faculty, even over email?

I remember a client who had few friends in high school but was relatively happy. But when she arrived at college, her anxiety really took over. After the initial excitement of orientation week, she retreated to her room and stopped socializing. She also stopped eating because she was anxious of how she looked walking around campus and having to see people in the dining hall. Her anxiety spiraled with the lack of eating and isolation.

Soon she stopped going to classes, and her RA [resident advisor] walked her over to my office for drop-in hours. She had a true case of social anxiety, not just the freshman jitters. With some reframing from a freshman CBT [cognitive behavioral therapy] group and some (very mild) exposure challenges, she had built a small supportive friend group by the end of the year.

—**Jeannie, therapist at a large Christian southern university**

My best friend 'came out' to me with social anxiety a few months into the school year. I'd actually begun to write them off as not wanting to hang out, and had stopped reaching out. It was so helpful for me as a friend to begin to understand that going out three nights a week, and meals with all new people three times a day, was just so hard for them. It wasn't that they didn't want to; it was just more effort. We talked about how to support them, and just decided we'd hang out less, and I'd try to remember to make sure there were other people around who they knew when we went out. They are grateful that I understood, and I was grateful that supporting them could be that simple. I mean, it's way more than that, but that there were some simple ways I could support them.

—**Amanda, friend of someone with social anxiety**

How Can I Manage Social Anxiety?

Unfortunately, to get better do have to get yourself out there and practice, like exposure therapy, but your therapist can help you do this at a pace that works for you. Mindfulness, relaxation practices, and CBT are very useful, and more general psychodynamic therapy can help you understand yourself in these situations as well. Medications like SSRIs, benzodiazepines, and beta blockers might help, too.

What Is Obsessive-Compulsive Disorder?

We've all heard someone say "I'm so OCD" as they clean their room or organize their notebook, and we had a sense of what that means: uptight, perfectionistic, fastidious, inflexible, neatnik, anal-retentive. And yet that's not exactly obsessive-compulsive disorder (OCD), which is a disruptive and excruciating issue with intrusive "obsessive" thoughts and compulsive behaviors (often about safety or health) that feel out of control and shameful. Many professionals feel that when someone casually describes themselves as OCD, not only are they not likely to have actual OCD but are doing a disservice to those really suffering.

OCD, like most mental illnesses, typically appears around the teen or young adult years. This is not because the stress of school causes OCD, although it can feel like it, but rather that college stress can trigger OCD in those students who are predisposed to it. Compared to other disorders, OCD is relatively rare, impacting around 1%–2% of the population, but it also tends to hide itself well.

Many of us, especially students, have our rituals and superstitions around studying or performances. Still others are uptight about certain things like germs, cleanliness, or neatness, and just about all of us have thoughts and worries about social situations or schoolwork, but these rarely cause much trouble or interfere with life. We may even have a sense of humor about them. Still others have weird thoughts and urges occasionally, a common one being wondering if they'll jump from a great height, but they don't feel actively suicidal.

But if you have or have seen real OCD up close, you will know all too well the repeated, unwanted thoughts and fears—also known as obsessions—which in turn can push someone to repetitive behaviors—also known as compulsions—to keep the obsessions in check. These obsessions and compulsions at extremes can really mess up your life.

What is especially frustrating are when those attempts to manage obsessions only increase your distress and anxiety, and you need more compulsions to ease the discomfort. However, despite efforts to ignore or get rid of the thoughts or urges, or doing compulsive acts to reduce obsessions, the obsessions keep coming back. This in turn leads to more ritualistic compulsions, and these set up the vicious cycle of OCD, which you may have already noticed often just gets worse over time.

OCD often centers on certain themes—for example, an excessive worry of getting contaminated by germs, or that you will harm yourself, or that you are a bad person because you have certain sexual desires. To ease your contamination fears, you might compulsively wash your hands to the point that they're sore and chapped, or for an amount of time that makes you late for class.

For an OCD diagnosis, you need to have obsessions, compulsions, or both, defined and described below. They also need to disrupt *at least an hour of your time each day* and last for a few weeks. We all obsess about a crush, frantically relive and relitigate interactions or tests we wish we'd done differently, but when it happens regularly, and over a few weeks, then we start to worry.

What Are Obsessions?

Obsessions are recurrent and persistent thoughts, images, urges, or impulses that are intrusive and unwanted. They usually cause significant anxiety, distress, or shame.

Harvard psychologist Dr. Brian Ott says, "Patients describe it like having a song in your head that won't go away; it's there all the time, the same thought popping in again and again."

Typically people know the thoughts aren't logical and react with repetitive actions to try and stop them, called compulsions. To build on Dr. Ott's metaphor, the compulsion is like listening to a song to get it out of your head, but with OCD that only works in the short term; the song keeps coming back. Because this is all happening in your mind, others may not recognize that what is happening for you is confusing, overwhelming, or even downright terrifying.

Red Flags for You

- [ ] *Are you finding it difficult to concentrate because of weird or scary thoughts that won't stop?*
- [ ] *Do you replay conversations again and again, worried that the other person has judged you or you said something bad?*
- [ ] *Is it hard to focus on what you need to, such as a final paper, because of your worries?*

Red Flags for Your Support Network

- [ ] *Do you notice the person distracted or agitated? Do they seem unfocused or "not totally present," maybe thinking distressing thoughts?*
- [ ] *Do they share worries that seem particularly "out there" that no amount of reassurance helps?*

What Are Compulsions?

Compulsions are repetitive behaviors. For example, these may present as excessive hand washing, rituals such as ordering school supplies in a certain pattern, or repeatedly going back and checking your door to see if it's locked despite having already checked if you locked it. They may also be mental actions such as counting objects, or even looking for patterns or repeating words or numbers silently. Compulsions exist to reduce or manage worry or distress, and you may imagine that they could even prevent something from happening.

Typically, the obsessions or compulsions suck up time and energy, for at least an hour a day, which lead to academic and social difficulties, in addition to shame and stigma. Most students recognize their OCD beliefs and behaviors in moments of clarity. But for many, and certainly in the moment, they feel very, very real and overwhelming.

continued

Red Flags for You

☐ *Are you having trouble getting things done because of rituals?*

☐ *Do you rush back to your dorm, minutes after you have left, to check to see that you have locked the door, and then do it again and again?*

☐ *Are you spending a lot of time in the bathroom washing your hands, and are your roommates complaining about the amount of soap you are using?*

☐ *Are your friends commenting on your behavior, or are you hiding it more and more?*

☐ *Is it taking up more than an hour of your time?*

Red Flags for Your Support Network

☐ *Are you noticing friends obsessing about things being arranged a certain way, or cleaning and disinfecting, in ways that make them run late or catch up with you later?*

☐ *Are they constantly worried or even checking if they left things unlocked, or the oven on, and so forth?*

☐ *Do you feel like you are constantly reassuring them or waiting for them to "double check" things?*

Checking your door lock at night and washing your hands after working in the garden are sensible behaviors. Even double checking or extra wash and rinse can be an extra measure. But doing these behaviors five or ten or twenty times in a row means that it is time for a different approach to the situation—passively focusing on the thoughts instead of actively trying to avoid or neutralize them through actions which will never be enough.

—**Brian Ott, author and faculty member
at William James College and Harvard Medical School**

What Are Some Different Types of OCD?

So far we've reviewed the general principles and symptoms of OCD. But there are many specific ways it manifests, and we thought we'd share a few of the more common ones. Here are a few examples of more common OCD types, but there are many more.

- **Fear of saying the wrong thing.** You might avoid social situations or commenting online out of a fear of blurting out something stupid, offensive, racist, or ignorant. You might also worry that bad things will happen if you say certain things. We've met students who spend hours scrolling back through their comments online just to make sure they didn't accidentally "like" something.

- **Harm OCD.** These are overwhelming feelings that you are going to harm yourself or someone else. Sometimes it's a fear that while you're slicing a bagel, you'll have an impulse to stab yourself or someone else. Or that on a boat or a height, you'll have the urge to jump. While many people have intrusive thoughts like these occasionally, for some people they really interfere with daily things like, well, being on boats and eating bagels. Kidding aside, many students are worried these intrusive thoughts will lead to hospitalization—a good practitioner knows the differences between these OCD thoughts and actual risk to self or others.

- **Relationship OCD.** This is when you have intrusive and distressing thoughts about your feelings of attraction or love for your romantic partner. We all worry about this from time to time, but is it dominating your life, messing up your relationships, or distracting you for hours a week for weeks on end?

- **Body-focused, or somatic, OCD.** This is a seemingly unending hyper-awareness of various bodily sensations. Your thoughts may be drawn to normal bodily functions such as breathing, blinking, swallowing, body position, joint pains, and itching, and even worries about concussions and tinnitus.

- **Trichotillomania.** This is related to OCD and includes symptoms like persistent hair pulling, skin picking, and other compulsions that aren't full-blown self-harm. Many people have nervous tics, and pick their cuticles or zits, but trichotillomania is when it tips into affecting your life and appearance in negative ways. We've seen bleeding, scars, or large bald patches on people's heads. Medication and CBT can help a lot.

- **Body dysmorphic disorder.** This is its own form of OCD and involves the obsessions focusing on appearance or aspects of appearance to the degree that causes distress and disfunction. Body dysmorphic disorder differs from an eating disorder or other forms of body image issues.

Regardless of the type of OCD you struggle with, the following three components are generally present: triggers, avoidance, and reassurance. But what do they all mean?

A *trigger* is the event or situation that sets off the obsessional worry; this can be a place, a person, an object, an interaction, an emotion, or even a thought. For example, you have the obsessional thought that assignments issued by your professor need to include certain words and contain a specific number of words, and that if you can't use the words, or your essay is too short, that you will fail the course. In this circumstance, being assigned homework is the trigger that prompts the obsessions and compulsions.

Avoidance is a common compulsion, as is the behavior of avoiding the people, places, or objects that you feel trigger an OCD cycle in an attempt to prevent distress, or to prevent hours of wasted time doing the compulsions. People will avoid objects, places, or people that they fear trigger their OCD.

For example, if you have a checking compulsion, and go back and check to see if your room door is locked, you might avoid leaving the dorm. Or, if you have an obsessional thought that you might stab someone, you might avoid having any sharp object in your room, even objects necessary for your class assignments, such as scissors. If you have a fear of germs, you might avoid taking a class in microbiology, even though you want to attend medical or nursing school.

Reassurance is the act of seeking certainty that your fear is not a reality. You might reach out to friends or family members, or search the news to make sure that some disaster that happened in the world wasn't your fault. Or you might check in with a loved one to see whether because you didn't do some behavior a specific number of times, that something bad didn't happen to them. Another obsessional fear that can lead to reassurance seeking in college is to allay the fear that your romantic partner no longer cares for you, or that something you said is the only thing that they can think about and that they are now upset because of what you said. Unfortunately, excessive reassurance seeking often only pushes people away.

Red Flags for You

- [ ] *Are you seeking reassurance from others a lot of the time?*
- [ ] *Even when you have been reassured, do you go back and check again?*
- [ ] *Do you feel as if you can never get enough reassurance?*

Red Flags for Your Support Network

- [ ] *Do your friends and loved ones comment on your need for reassurance?*
- [ ] *Do they say you worry too much?*
- [ ] *Do they wonder why you keep asking them the same questions over and over?*

I know this isn't nice, but I had a neighbor in my apartment building during college who had OCD and we'd watch her, it was really sad actually. Every morning I'd wake up to these weird sounds and footsteps, and finally one day I watched out my keyhole. She'd pull the door, check the knob twenty times, then walk away, sometimes down the stairs, then stop, then walk back, check it again, and would do that again and again. Sometimes I'd hear her come back four or five times. She never did it when anyone else was around, and I know I should not have spied, but it was fascinating.

—**Aimee, college graduate now teaching history**

I found a combo of medication and cognitive behavioral therapy most helpful for my OCD. I would have thoughts that I accidentally liked something on social media, and just kept going back and scrolling again and again, and then worried when I was checking that I had accidentally liked something. It sounds so stupid and was so embarrassing, that was just one of my obsession/compulsions.

—**Erica, junior at a medium-sized university**

Treating OCD

So what's the best way to treat OCD? Typically a combination of a stricter version of CBT with a specialist can help a lot, and often some SSRI medications can make a difference as well.

What Is Trauma? And What Is Posttraumatic Stress Disorder?

What Trauma Isn't

We've all heard folks throw diagnoses around casually, for instance, maybe when a friend bombed an exam and told you they were depressed, when more accurately, they were disappointed. That classmate who confessed that their "OCD" study plan failed them is not right either. By the same token, telling others that you were traumatized by the bad grade is not an accurate use of the word *trauma*, no matter how bad you feel.

So, Then, What Is Trauma?

Mental health professionals mostly agree that psychological trauma is an event or situation that results in physical or psychological harm. It is an extremely distressing event that is often life threatening or otherwise threatening to your body or your sense of self. Many consider emotional traumas and neglect, or being close to a traumatic event, to be traumas as well. The word comes from the more medical term of physical trauma or injury, and sometimes the two go hand in hand. Let's explain more.

What Are Traumatic Events?

The most common traumatic events for students include a physical or sexual assault, or experiencing a life-threatening accident, illness, or injury. Although women are somewhat less likely to experience traumatic events overall (Norris, 2002), they are more vulnerable to sexual assault and childhood sexual abuse than men (Tolin, 2006). For instance, nearly one in five women has been raped, according to extensive surveys (Black, 2011). Trauma can impact your mental, physical, social, and spiritual well-being.

These days, a tragic number of current college students have lived through incidents of gun violence. Others grew up in traumatic environments with domestic violence and abuse in the home, and others in their neighborhoods or countries of origin. Many military veteran students have combat-related trauma. And certainly far too many students have been sexually assaulted or harassed before and during college. Other traumas may include unrelenting bullying, as well as racial discrimination and other forms of identity based trauma.

What are the Emotional Consequences of Traumatic Events?

There is no one emotional response to a traumatic event. As clinicians like to say, "If you've met one person with a trauma history, you've met one person with a trauma history." Still, the type of traumatic event matters, and your response may be very different than others who survived the exact same traumatic event. You might feel nervous, helpless, sad, or afraid. You may feel numb, almost emotionless. You might feel angry and irritable and snap easily. You might feel guilty or responsible for whatever bad things happened, or even for surviving when others had it worse. You might lose trust in other people and feel that you have to control things because no one else seems to be responsible. You might feel very alone and abandoned by the people you were closest to and, in this context, have no desire for intimacy with others. All of these, as they say, are normal reactions to an abnormal event.

What are Childhood Traumas and Adverse Childhood Experiences?

While trauma can happen on campus, many students come to school with a history of trauma. Recently, researchers have created a list of 10 types of traumatic childhood events known as adverse childhood experiences (ACEs) that contribute to difficulties in health, mental health, relationships, and learning later in life.

Take a look over this list and see if anything resonates for you, people you know, or even your own family.

- Physical abuse
- Emotional abuse
- Sexual abuse
- Physical neglect
- Emotional neglect
- Mental illness in household
- Divorce or separation of parents, or abandonment by a parent
- Witnessing domestic violence
- Substance abuse
- Incarcerated family member

You may look at this list and resonate with a number of these and start to worry there's something wrong with you. But remember, the list does not take into account protective factors that outweigh these, such as trustworthy adults, a strong sense of community and belonging (like a team, club, or church), a sense of purpose (like academic drive or community service), and a number of other factors that can help prevent complications to your mental health. That also means that it's important to try to find these protective factors in college as soon as you can, which we discuss more in "Finding and Building a Network" on Chapter 6.

It's important to know that just because you have ACEs does not mean that you have posttraumatic stress disorder (PTSD) or are doomed to develop mental health issues. ACEs just increase the risk of those things. In fact, many people have ACEs and don't just survive but thrive, especially when they start therapy. So if you've made it to college after a high ACE score, you're clearly doing many things right and have been for a long time. Still, some of those survival mechanisms may be ones to let go of now that you are in a safer environment.

I learned about ACEs in a training I had for a volunteer thing I was doing between junior and senior year. I gave myself the quiz and literally had almost every single one. And suddenly so much made sense about the way I was getting into bad relationships with people, doing too many drugs the first few years in college. When I got back to campus, I started counseling with the eight free sessions the school offered, and started to understand myself so much better.

—D'Nora, college graduate who is now an elementary school teacher

How Common Is Posttraumatic Stress Disorder?

Before diving deeper, it might be helpful, even inspiring, to know the following: Many people experience traumatic events in their life, but the majority of them do *not* go on to develop PTSD. In fact, only about 7% of people get PTSD over the course of their lives, and again, this hits women harder than men, at about a 5:1 ratio.[4] Research (Benjet, 2016) shows that 70% of all of us will experience at least one trauma in our lifetime, and more than 30% will experience four or more, but most do not develop PTSD. This means that the majority of people who experience traumatic events do not go on to develop full-blown PTSD, even if the traumatic event has some of the consequences we mentioned earlier.

So What Is PTSD?

Before someone is diagnosed with PTSD, they need to have experienced a trauma. This can be a direct traumatic experience, such as being the victim of a violent act. Or it can be witnessing other people undergoing a traumatic event, such as being with a friend as they overdosed. Or it can be learning that a close friend or relative was exposed to a traumatic event, like hearing about a brutal sexual assault.

After the event, there are four groups of symptoms that emerge:

1. Intrusive memories of the event
2. Avoidance of people, places, and anything that reminds you of the traumatic event
3. Negative changes in your thinking and mood
4. Changes in physical and emotional reactions

Intrusive memories

These are ways in which you reexperience the traumatic situation and can include the following:

- Upsetting memories of the event
- Flashbacks/intrusive memories or reexperiencing parts of the event
- Nightmares of the event
- Overwhelmed with negative emotions when reminded of the trauma
- Strong physical and physiological reactions whenever reminded of the trauma

Red Flags for You

☐ *Do powerful thoughts of the event pop into your head, or do you have feelings that flood your body in overwhelming ways?*

☐ *Do small things "trigger" a massive physiological response in your mind or body?*

☐ *Are you unable to, or even scared of, falling asleep because you have nightmares?*

☐ *Do you ever feel the event happening again in your senses?*

☐ *Do you find yourself thinking over and over about the situation?*

Red Flags for Your Support Network

☐ *Does the person struggle with sleep or nightmares, looking tired or complaining about sleep?*

☐ *Do they have a short fuse or become triggered by small things?*

☐ *Do they seem to "disappear" into themselves, dissociate, and struggle to "snap out of it" in a way that's not like ADHD?*

☐ *Do they talk over and over about the situation, or strongly avoid talking about it?*

Avoidance

This means, literally, avoiding certain situations and includes the following:

- Avoiding thinking or talking to others about the event
- Avoiding people, places, or activities that are reminders
- Using substances, behaviors, or self-harm to avoid or blunt emotions associated with the traumatic event.

continued

Red Flags for You

☐ *Do you avoid thinking about the event?*
☐ *Do you notice not wanting to talk to people when they bring up the situation?*
☐ *Do you avoid people, places, or things that might be associated with the trauma?*
☐ *Do you use behaviors or substances to escape your emotions and blunt any triggers?*

Red Flags for Your Support Network

☐ *Does the person isolate in their room more or avoid certain places?*
☐ *Are there topics of conversation that seem unrelated to the trauma, but they change the subject, get flustered, or leave altogether?*
☐ *Are there people, places, and things they seem to avoid that might be related?*
☐ *Are they using drugs or self-harm, particularly during triggering moments?*

Negative changes in thinking and mood

These are particularly evident if you used to be a more positive person.

- Negative thinking about yourself, such as blame and shame, or negative thoughts about others, especially about trust
- Hopelessness about the future, asking yourself, "What's the point?"
- Memory issues that make you doubt yourself
- Disconnection from older relationships, difficulty forming new ones
- Lack of interest in usual activities
- Difficulty in experiencing positive emotions
- Feeling emotionally numb, or not even real

Red Flags for You

☐ *Do you notice changes in your personality—that you used to be a more optimistic person but are pessimistic and cynical, or rarely feel positive emotions?*
☐ *Have you stopped planning for the future and wonder, "What's the point?"*
☐ *Have you stopped enjoying the things that used to make you happy?*
☐ *Do you blame yourself or feel guilty about more things, especially the trauma?*
☐ *Do you feel numb or disconnected from people?*

Red Flags for Your Support Network

☐ *Do they seem suddenly different?*
☐ *Have they dropped their clubs, activities, and previous priorities?*
☐ *Do they isolate more from people or have more conflicts?*
☐ *Do they seem down, out of it, or disconnected from themselves?*

Changes in physical and emotional reactions (also called arousal symptoms)

This is what people often talk about in terms of trauma being in the body or nervous system. They include the following:

- Easily startled or frightened, like when a phone rings or a door slams
- Always on guard for danger, looking over your shoulder, insisting that a friend accompany you, always keeping an eye on the door or another escape route
- Self-injury, substance misuse, and harmful behaviors like spending sprees to change how you feel or to feel less numb
- Trouble falling asleep, staying asleep, or waking up early with upsetting thoughts
- Trouble concentrating and focusing, which makes it particularly difficult if you are a student
- Feeling irritable and having episodic anger outbursts or even physically aggressive behavior
- Overwhelming guilt or shame, especially if sexual violence is the trauma
- Hot and cold flashes in the body; breath and heart rate changes when triggered

Red Flags for You

☐ *Are you not sleeping well, tossing and turning at night, with light sleep filled with anxious thoughts?*
☐ *Do you feel exhausted the next day because of poor sleep?*
☐ *Do you feel that you are to blame or feel guilty?*
☐ *Do you have trouble focusing and feel "foggy?"*
☐ *Do you feel "jumpier" or on edge?*
☐ *Are you "jumpier" than usual?*

I didn't realize that constantly being on edge, always scanning for danger, and jumping at the drop of a hat was a symptom of trauma. I was also having trouble

continued

focusing and then started to wonder about ADHD. I thought I was just being safe! My best friend told to ask my therapist, and it was really helpful to understand that and work through a car wreck my friends and I had been through in high school.

Jesse, freshman accounting major from Texas

Red Flags for Your Support Network

- ☐ *Do they seem jumpy, snippy, irritable, or even aggressive?*
- ☐ *Are they much more worried about safety—locking doors, showing excessive caution about car safety, or never being alone at social events?*
- ☐ *Is sleep and exhaustion an issue?*
- ☐ *Are grades falling along with focus?*
- ☐ *Are you seeing an uptick in self-harm, substance use, or other avoidance behaviors?*

These symptoms generally point to a trauma, stress, or even PTSD response. And there are many things that can help—talk therapy, art therapy, eye movement desensitization reprocessing, support groups, activism, and sometimes even medication can help settle the nervous system as well.

So If That's PTSD, What's Acute Stress Disorder?

Technically, PTSD doesn't get diagnosed until a month after the event. Before that, it's known as acute stress disorder.

What About Sexual Violence and Sexual Trauma?

For too many students, sexual violence is an experience that can occur in high school or college. This can include rape, assault, or sexual harassment, even just unwanted sexual attention, all of which can feel disempowering, shameful, and traumatic. The likelihood of experiencing sexual violence in the first and second semesters is higher than the rest of college,[5] but it remains high throughout. Whether it is verbal or physical, it can leave lasting, painful damage that affects feelings of physical and emotional safety, and intimate relationships, and it can severely impact mental health. That's even before the academic and social challenges that can come after sexual violence. If you or a friend has experienced sexual violence, we hope that this section offers an idea of where and how to start the healing process.

What Should I Do If I've Experienced Sexual Violence?

- Get yourself or friend to safety—away from the party, house, or dorm, and to a safe room where there is some privacy. Not easy to find, we know. You might go directly to the infirmary or public safety.
- Remember self-care. You just experienced something scary and awful. Nothing can fix it right now or change that it happened, but what would make you feel even 5% better right now? Whether it's talking to a friend, gaming, listening to music, journaling, or something else, take a small step toward caring for yourself right now.
- Consider medical attention. It's important to get checked out, not just if you later file a complaint, but, unfortunately for injury, sexually trans-mitted infections, potential pregnancy, and so forth. There are medica-tions that can be taken right away to prevent pregnancy or infection. The infirmary or hospital also may offer to take physical evidence and a statement, what's called a "rape kit," if there's an investigation later. Unfortunately, while the first thing someone wants to do is shower, this is not a good idea because it may also wash away evidence. And, while challenging, write down anything you can remember.
- There is a good chance that your college's mental health center, Title IX office, or sexual assault coordinator will have guidance on your options moving forward. Every school is different, but we encourage you to familiarize yourself with the procedures early, in case you or a friend does need support. You might also want to reach out to local crisis cen-ters or see if local police departments have witness advocates, who might know about university policies from a different perspective. Whether you'd like to take any kind of action against the perpetrator or not, know-ing what options you have will help you feel empowered and regain some sense of control, after a trauma that has left you feeling disempowered and out of control.
- Even if you end up not pressing charges on campus or with the police, at least you will know what resources are available. Are you feeling uncer-tain about how to proceed? You don't need to decide right now anyway, and you have a lot of time to call a hotline, talk it out with a trusted friend or family member, consult a mental health professional, or journal about

the situation to find some clarity. Rarely is there a rush to make a decision on anything but the physical evidence collection.

- Seek support and find community. Whether it's extra sessions with your mental health professional, time away from classes or school, joining a group for survivors of sexual violence, joining an activist group, or reading a comforting book, try to take one step to receive more support or understanding. Processing trauma alone can be incredibly isolating, so try to find a way to connect.

- Do one extra comforting thing per day. It's important that you ramp up your self-care activities at this time. Make a list of 10 things that you can do that help you feel safe in your body, relaxed, or even slightly more peaceful. Don't know where to start? Review Chapter 4 on self-care. Whether it be at the start of your day, between classes, or before bedtime, see if you can take even five minutes to do something sweet for yourself to get through this time.

- At some point, perhaps not today, consider reporting what happened. There are complaints you can make to the school, as well as to the police, and these are different processes. Campus resources should hopefully be able to help you understand what your rights are with regard to the police, as well as on campus in terms of requesting accommodations for safety, academics, and even housing. You can also request "stay away" orders to the person in question, if you want them.

And even though you've been told and learned so much about how it's not your fault, it may still feel like it is. That's how rape culture is internalized, and it might take a lot of work to undo it in yourself. Be extra gentle with yourself at this time and seek out support to work through any of those ideas or thoughts that might be present.

What Should I Do If a Friend Has Experienced Sexual Violence?

- **Listen, affirm, and reflect.** Your friend has just experienced one of the hardest things someone can go through. If you take the time to give them your full attention, empathize with their feelings, and reflect back what you're hearing, it can probably mean the world. You don't have to be a trained listener to make someone feel heard and understood. Just be available and let them know that you understand that they might feel scared, overwhelmed, frozen, angry, or distraught.

- **Share resources and connect your friend.** You can share our resources or any that you may know about on campus or in the community. You could even do some research on your friend's behalf or with them to see what's available. See if your friend would like help making phone calls, sending emails, or transportation. Ensure that they make a connection to some kind of resource so that you know that they're getting help. Remember, too, to take good care of yourself during this time.
- **Check in.** It means a lot when a friend checks in after going through a tough time. Send them a text to ask them how they're doing. Make plans to get lunch or watch a movie together. Give them a hug. Or even better, ask your friend how you can best support them through this and try to meet their needs as much as your capacity allows. What often hurts the most is feeling abandoned by friends after sexual violence occurs.

Resources

- Online chat: online.rainn.org
- Hotline: National Sexual Assault Hotline (1-800-656-4673)
- Books
  - *The Rape Recovery Handbook: Step-by-Step Help for Survivors of Sexual Assault* by Aphrodite T. Matsakis
  - *Growing Beyond Survival: A Self-Help Toolkit for Managing Traumatic Stress* by Elizabeth G. Vermilyea
  - *You Can Help: A Guide for Family & Friends of Survivors of Sexual Abuse and Assault* by Rebecca Street
- Websites
  - National Sexual Violence Resource Center (https://www.nsvrc.org/)
  - Forge (For survivors in Trans Community) (https://forge-forward.org/)
  - Love Is Respect (for survivors in unsafe relationships) (https://www.loveisrespect.org/)
  - 1in6 (for survivors who are men) (https://1in6.org/)

I didn't realize the impact that the sexual assault that I experienced had on me. I thought it wasn't that bad because he just touched me inappropriately at a party and I wasn't raped. But it made me hypervigilant. I was always on edge. I didn't connect the dots until I started therapy. Doing somatic exercises helped me feel safe in my body again. I learned how to slow down and accept that what happened to me was traumatic, even if it could've been worse.

—Samira, 21, junior at a large southern university

My daughter felt so broken after she was raped. I didn't know what to do. . . . It's a mom's worst nightmare. Her grades suffered, and everything just got bad. I tried to encourage her to take the rest of the semester off, and luckily she agreed. We were able to focus on helping her feel safe and whole again without the distractions of school and any of the triggering people or environments there. When she returned, she had her best semester yet. Sometimes she still struggles, but she has the tools she needs to get through those times.

—**Jennifer, 46, parent**

Many students don't even realize they are the survivors of sexual violence, whether harassment or assault, until months or even years later. Harassment and acquaintance rape are particularly insidious in this way. We live in a world in which these things are minimized and kept hidden and shameful, in many senses even from ourselves. Students should know that its never too late to get get help, even if time has passed or something occurred in high school or off campus.

—**David, therapist at a large, private Midwestern university**

In Conclusion

Adjustment, anxiety, and trauma are real, and they are simultaneously overdiagnosed and overlooked. As you learn more about them, we hope that you can understand more clearly the specifics of the disorders themselves and the treatments for them. For those who have experienced or have been close to another's experience of sexual violence, we hope that this chapter helps you navigate the process with as much ease and care as possible.

Chapter 11
Mood Disorders and Psychosis

Certain mood disorders and psychotic disorders can fall under the category of more severe mental health issues that are more likely to be dangerous in terms of suicide or other behaviors, and more likely to require medication or sometimes hospitalization for safety. While there are many milder forms of mood disorders that are very common, at their most extreme they need immediate intervention. Understanding the differences between depression and dysthymia, types of bipolar disorders, and less frequently, types of psychosis, is important for getting the right help at the right time.

What Is Major Depression?

Depression and mood disorders are the second most common mental health issue facing college students, after anxiety disorders. These days, young adults have higher rates of depression than older generations, with some estimates as high as 20% of young adults experiencing depression, female-identified people about twice as likely as male to experience depression, and higher rates in mixed-race people.[1]

Of course, everyone has felt even extreme ups and downs, especially in the roller coaster of college. But major depression is that flat and down feeling (or in guys it's often grumpiness and irritability), but those symptoms usually last beyond a few weeks.

Adjusting to freshman year or even coming back from break is its own challenge, too, so you might think about a bit more than just a few weeks. Life in college is very different than the real world—that's why college can simultaneously be so amazing and so challenging. You'll notice many symptoms can look like adjustment issues and homesickness, so you want to watch that these symptoms are still occurring deeper into the year than just the first few weeks back at school.

You'll probably notice many symptoms might be symptoms of other conditions as well, and that's why it is so important to check in with a professional who can determine what is going on, whether it is depression or something else. In fact, many folks may experience mood changes due to hormonal changes, whether that's just your body (at extremes this can be premenstrual dysphoric disorder [PMDD]), your birth control, or hormones you may be taking if you are trans. Other issues like thyroid and other health problems may be impacting you as well, so get checked out by your regular doctor.

Look over this list of symptoms. You may not relate to every one of them for yourself or someone you care about, but a few may jump out at you.

What Are the Symptoms of Major Depression?

Bodily and Physical Symptoms

Aches, pains, cramps, and digestive problems that don't respond to standard treatment

Red Flags for You

- [ ] *Have you noticed more medical issues, upset stomach, aches and pains, or even just physical discomforts lately?*

Red Flags for Your Support Network

- [ ] *Is the person complaining about pains or discomfort?*
- [ ] *Are they taking trips to the doctor and not finding anything particularly wrong?*

Exhaustion

Red Flags for You

- [ ] *College is exhausting, and getting decent sleep is almost impossible. But overall, do the usual things like socializing and academics seem to take more energy than they used to?*

☐ *One student told us that doing anything, even just getting out of bed and getting dressed, takes her twice as much effort when she is depressed.*

Red Flags for Your Support Network

☐ *Are they going out less and getting less done than usual?*
☐ *Do they seem tired all the time and lethargic?*
☐ *Do they not have the energy to do the things they used to?*

Overeating or undereating with 5% weight gain or loss

Red Flags for You

☐ *Again, this is hard when so many students gain the notorious "freshman 15," while others can't find food they like at school and lose a few pounds. A better question is: Are there significant changes in your appetite?*
☐ *Is your appetite more or less than usual?*
☐ *Or perhaps you notice yourself eating mindlessly to cope?*
☐ *Or losing your appetite altogether?*

Red Flags for Your Support Network

☐ *Do they have significant weight gain or weight loss, are they are eating a lot more or less than usual, skipping meals, or not eating much during meals?*

Insomnia, disrupted sleeping, or too much sleeping

Red Flags for You

☐ *Because sleep is hard at college, the question is really: Is it harder to fall or stay asleep?*
☐ *Do you wake up early from worry or negative thoughts?*
☐ *Or are you sleeping too much, struggling to get out of bed, or crawling back into bed to nap after class?*
☐ *It is also important to look at those regular nights, not just nights when you might have been drinking or using substances.*

Red Flags for Your Support Network

☐ *Do they complain about not sleeping well lately?*
☐ *Or do they oversleep or nap often despite also sleeping at night?*

continued

Psychomotor changes

Red Flags for You

- [ ] *Do you find yourself more physically agitated and fidgety than usual?*
- [ ] *On the other side, do you feel like you are moving and taking it more slowly lately?*

Red Flags for Your Support Network

- [ ] *Have you noticed the person is more fidgety lately, or conversely, moving and speaking more slowly in recent weeks?*
- [ ] *Do they take longer than usual to get things done?*

Psychological Symptoms

Feeling guilty, feeling like a bad person

Red Flags for You

- [ ] *How is your self-esteem recently?*
- [ ] *Most of us feel a little guilty when we mess up, but are you feeling guilty or worthless over minor things that you used to just get over?*
- [ ] *Do you feel like a bad person a lot of the time?*

Red Flags for Your Support Network

- [ ] *Do you notice this person putting themselves down and being harder on themselves more often, over seemingly small things?*

Feeling hopeless or pessimistic

Red Flags for You

- [ ] *Do things like life, college, friendships, schoolwork, and the future seem pointless?*
- [ ] *Is seeing the positive lately a huge challenge?*
- [ ] *Do you feel bad about yourself, the world, and the future?*

Red Flags for Your Support Network

☐ *Do you notice growing pessimism and negative comments from the person?*

Sad, empty, depressed, or anxious feelings

Red Flags for You

☐ *Are you crying often and not sure why?*
☐ *Are you feeling sad, empty, or numb?*
☐ *Are you worried more than usual?*
☐ *Or do you feel sad and wish you could cry but can't?*

Red Flags for Your Support Network

☐ *Do you notice this person crying, fighting back tears, or looking down or anxious?*
☐ *Do you notice a significant change in their mood, more down and worried?*
☐ *Do they talk about feeling empty or numb and don't know why?*

Thoughts of death, thoughts of suicide, suicide attempts (more about suicide on Chapter 1)

Red Flags for You

☐ *Have you been thinking about death?*
☐ *Do you have thoughts or plans to, or even tried, to hurt or kill yourself?*
☐ *Have you found yourself wondering about feeling relief if you're gone, and/or how or whether others will feel sad or impacted in some way by your death?*
☐ *Have you found yourself in some way preparing to say goodbye or leave things behind to others?*

Red Flags for Your Support Network

☐ *Has the person talked about death or dying more, or that no one would care if they disappeared or died?*
☐ *Have they made suicide attempts in the past or talked about plans, even vague, to end their life?*
☐ *Have they been giving away things that are important to them, as if they know they will die?*

continued

What are the Social and Behavioral Symptoms?

Loss of interest in the usual activities

Red Flags for You

- [ ] *Do your friends and classes interest you less?*
- [ ] *Are grades even in your favorite classes slipping?*
- [ ] *What about your clubs, jobs, internships and volunteer work?*
- [ ] *What about your favorite books, shows, and websites?*
- [ ] *Is your sex drive down?*

Red Flags for Your Support Network

- [ ] *Has the person been isolating more, seen you less often, been less involved in things, and less "present" even when there physically?*
- [ ] *Are they often not enjoying things they used to—shows, video games, and parties now seem boring and so forth?*
- [ ] *Have they quit a number of activities they used to enjoy?*

Irritability, restlessness

Red Flags for You

- [ ] *Do people and minor situations get on your nerves more quickly?*
- [ ] *Do you get bored more often?*
- [ ] *Are you less able to hang in with activities or interactions with others that used to come easily to you?*

Red Flags for Your Support Network

- [ ] *Does the person seem more irritable, abrupt, and "short" with others?*
- [ ] *Do they quit things more quickly?*
- [ ] *Are they making more self-deprecating remarks with ever darker and more cynical humor lately?*

How many of these can you relate to now, or ever? Even a few symptoms lasting for more than a few weeks can be considered dysthymia, a milder form of depression for which therapy and medication can help. We'll talk more about that in the next section.

Which ones would you consider your red flags or early warning signs? Which ones do you feel comfortable asking other people to keep an eye on for you?

I had depression on and off through high school, and was managing it pretty well with weekly therapy sessions and medication. For me, depression felt like a heavy weight on my chest that made it hard to get out of bed, to get to school, to do anything. It was manageable at college up until my junior year when it suddenly came back in force while I was studying in Copenhagen, where it got super dark. I had to make some adjustments like being sure I was up and out when it was light out, making sure I got more exercise and so forth, and back in touch via Zoom with my home therapist. The seasonal thing is very real, and especially if you're from a warm light place, moving back east or up north to school can be tough on depression.

—Amir, college graduate who is now a sound engineer

As parents, we worry about everything. And Santi just sounded different in his calls. His voice was flat, he always seemed tired, his grades were falling, and he didn't like his friends. He'd come home for break and stay in his pajamas all day, which seemed maybe normal for a college kid? But he talked a lot about transferring during most of his freshman and part of his sophomore year. But sophomore year he called and told us it was depression, and that he'd started seeing a counselor on campus. We were even more worried at first, but soon it was clear that the counseling was really helpful to him and I feel like we owe his life to the campus wellness center.

—Rita, parent of Santi, who was sociology major
and is now a successful activist

I just cried every day and could not figure out why. At first I thought I was home-sick. But after months of it, my best friend from home told my brother, who told my parents. I was definitely pissed at first, but in retrospect clearly I needed help. My parents made me an appointment with my doctor from home over break, and actually, you know what? It was my birth control. When I changed my birth control, my depression got so much better.

—Olivia, college graduate now working on her master's degree in history

What Is Seasonal Affective Disorder?

Seasonal affective disorder (SAD) is when depression symptoms arise or worsen during the fall and winter as days become shorter and darker. About 5% of the population appears to get SAD, with it lasting about 40% of the year in the winter months; it is four times as common in those identifying as female.[2] Not surprisingly, it's worse in northern climates than southern ones in North America and Europe. It's thought that it might have something to do with exposure to sunlight or a lack thereof. Many students are awake late and sleep later than the rest of the world, which can worsen the amount of time spent in sunlight. You might want to consider waking up earlier, getting an ultraviolet "happy lamp," or trying vitamin D supplements if SAD impacts you. It may also come as a surprise to students who attend college further north than where they are from, when the days are particularly short and cold in the fall and winter, that their mood is seriously impacted by the dark, the cold, and the time inside.

What Is Persistent Depressive Disorder or Dysthymia?

Similar to depression is what used to be called dysthymia and is now called persistent depressive disorder (PDD). It basically describes a milder but longer-lasting form of what we think of as depression. It's very real, and it can be very debilitating, even if it's considered "milder" than depression. About 2.5% of people experience PDD in their lives, according to the National Institute of Mental Health, again more common in those identifying as women.[3]

Basically, it means the person has a depressed mood most of the day, for most days of the week, without more than a few months break for at least two years. In a sense, it's a lighter, but longer kind of depression. Take a look back at the depression symptoms. Dysthymia needs to include two of the following:

- Overeating or undereating with 5% weight gain or loss (see above symptom in depression section)
- Insomnia, disrupted sleeping, or too much sleeping (see above symptom in depression section)
- Feeling exhausted or having much less energy (see above symptom in depression section)

- Low self-esteem (see above symptom in depression section)
- Feeling hopeless or pessimistic (see above symptom in depression section)

Poor Concentration or Difficulty Making Decisions

Red Flags for You

☐ *Do you have difficulty deciding on a major, study abroad, jobs, parties, and so on?*
☐ *Is this more from a sense of overwhelm and exhaustion than feeling like too many good choices?*
☐ *Do you have difficulty focusing for long periods of time?*
☐ *(Note this is a symptom of many things. It can also be hard to focus because nothing seems very interesting.)*

Red Flags for Your Support Network

☐ *Does this person not do things because they can't decide, or miss opportunities or blow deadlines because they can't decide or focus?*

During orientation, I cried every single day because I was so homesick. I couldn't have fun and make new friends. Also everyone was from a private school which was a shock and like a year older than me at least. It was very weird trying to form relationships. No one is from the South at my school so no one understood me. A lot of my unhealthy habits were distractions from how I was feeling. When I came home from winter break, I realized that I wasn't taking care of myself. When I went back to school, I started a habit tracker. I would journal, go on walks, and listen to wellness podcasts. I also make it a priority to go outside and be in the sun, and get out of my dorm room. Then I can be healthy and functional.

—Ayodele, sophomore at a small liberal arts college

My son was getting so negative about everything and I got really concerned. He was always so joyful and present as a teenager, so it freaked me out when he went to college and started to get so pessimistic. I would try to talk to him, but he didn't really open up. What really helped was when I visited him at school and met some of his friends. I spoke to them privately about my concerns and some of them shared their concerns as well. I was able to get them to encourage him to try therapy and get out more. I know it can be hard for men to share their feelings, plus I'm his mom, so I get it and didn't take his guardedness personally. Getting his friends involved allowed me to still help him but in a way that he can receive it.

—Callie, parent of a student-athlete at a public university

How Should Dysthymia And Minor Depression Be Treated?

Dysthymia and major depression are both treatable with talk therapy and medications like selective serotonin reuptake inhibitors (SSRIs) and others. There also tends to be a lot of overlap between depression and anxiety. As far as talk therapies, it seems like it depends most on the individual whether cognitive behavioral or psychodynamic therapies are most helpful, and often it's a combination of both.

What Are Manic and Bipolar Disorders?

Bipolar disorders, what used to be called "manic depression," are when moods swing between extreme highs and lows over the course of a few days or weeks. Now, everyone cycles between highs and lows, and all the social and relationships drama and excitement and all the academic demands of college mean a lot of cycling between "I aced the test" and "I lost my #1 bid." But true bipolar cycles are often unrelated to external events and change on their own. They are also dangerous, and they hit male- and female-identified students equally, with about 4.4% of people experiencing bipolar in their lifetime, and the average time it begins is at about age 25.[4] Again, sorting out what's a standard (and often unhealthy) college lifestyle and what's actually a bipolar disorder is tough, so let's look at the symptoms of so-called manic episodes, the extreme highs.

What Are Manic Episodes?

Manic episodes are distinct periods of abnormally and persistently elevated, expansive, or irritable mood, lasting at least a week with at least three of the following symptoms:

Inflated Self-Esteem or Grandiosity

Red Flags for You

☐ *Do you suddenly feeling almost invincible (with risky behavior), feeling massive amounts of (unrealistic) confidence?*

☐ *These are really hard to be aware of in ourselves, and also they often feel so good that we don't want them to stop. This may include thinking you can pull off unrealistic academic or creative projects, do copious amounts of drugs, take big risks or bets, and so forth.*

Red Flags for Your Support Network

☐ *Does this person have massive and unrealistic overconfidence about their abilities, ideas, and capabilities, and unrealistic timelines to accomplish these things?*

Decreased Need for Sleep

Red Flags for You

☐ *Are you sleeping far less, or not at all, without getting tired?*

Red Flags for Your Support Network

☐ *Does this person stay up late or not sleep at all, often frantically doing unnecessary projects or activities without seeming tired the next day?*
☐ *This is not "pulling an all-nighter" to get schoolwork done or meet another deadline and then crashing the next day.*

Excessive Talking or "Pressured Speech"

Red Flags for You

☐ *Does your brain move faster than your words, like you can't get it all out?*
☐ *Are you interrupting others, not letting them get a word in edgewise?*
☐ *Do your ideas seem too interesting and important to not keep talking about?*

Red Flags for Your Support Network

☐ *Does this person talk nonstop, interrupting others, not letting others get a word in edgewise, and rapidly jumping from seemingly unrelated idea to idea, often talking about unrealistic or strange ideas and plans?*

continued

Racing Thoughts

Red Flags for You

☐ *Do you feel like your thoughts are moving too fast, like you can't keep up with your own ideas, like you can't get all your thoughts out in words or writing fast enough?*

Red Flags for Your Support Network

☐ *Does this person look distracted and speak rapidly, constantly scribbling down notes or voice memos for ideas that don't make much sense?*

Distractibility

Red Flags for You

☐ *Do you start big projects and not finish them, rapidly change things like paper topics and social calendars, and are generally distracted, but far more than the usual indecision?*

Red Flags for Your Support Network

☐ *Does this person look distractedly around the room, changing conversation topics, changing social plans and groups rapidly, switching academic topics, starting and not finishing (often too big) projects, "biting off more than they can chew"?*
☐ *Do they chase down new campus activities, social clubs, interests, and people at the drop of a hat?*

Intense Goal-Directed Activity

Red Flags for You

☐ *Do you take on and go intense and deep on creative, academic, or business projects, often without sleep or breaks?*

Red Flags for Your Support Network

☐ *Does this person have excessive involvement in activities like unrealistic business plans and schemes, with religious intensity, coming up with elaborate plans for activities, parties, and events?*

Excessive Pleasurable Activities That Lead to Painful Consequences

Red Flags for You

☐ *Do you spend time and money, often beyond your means, on things that are just for fun or pleasure, not noticing or dealing with the financial, academic, and social consequences, or having huge denial about these?*

Red Flags for Your Support Network

☐ *Does this person binge on shopping, gambling, sex, luxury travel, substances, gaming, and more?*
☐ *Do lots of packages arrive?*
☐ *Do they disappear on spontaneous trips and so forth?*
☐ *This may look like or overlap with a substance abuse problem.*

So What Does This All Mean?

It's hard to describe a manic episode until you've experienced one or witnessed it. But we've seen clients rack up enormous shopping bills online as packages pile up in the campus mailroom, go on enormous spending sprees on strippers, or cheat on their partners for days on end before realizing the damage that's been caused to their partner and friendship circle. Many of these also look like addictions or compulsions, and are important to distinguish, although they certainly overlap. One father said to us about his son in the midst of a manic episode: "He was acting like he'd been up doing speed all night, but it was actually just a manic episode."

I remember a hallmate coming by freshman year and asking if I wanted to start a restaurant. It was fun, and we both love food and bullshitted around menu ideas into the night. I went to sleep, but the next morning she woke me up early talking a mile a minute and sharing a whole business PowerPoint plan, and had emailed her parents and the dean that she was dropping out of school. I suddenly realized she was serious, but delusional. I had thought we were just kind of kidding around. She had already maxed out her credit card buying supplies, and she asked me with an excited but straight face if I could ask my parents for a $50,000 loan to buy supplies, and it was then I realized something was seriously off. She later left school and we learned she was bipolar.

—Natasha, senior at a large private university

My brother FaceTimed me from Vegas one weekend, where he'd decided to use his credit card to fly himself and three friends first class for the weekend from Michigan! He booked a suite at some fancy hotel and was showing me the view. My parents were so upset, they do not have a ton of money and neither does my brother! He started doing that kind of crazy thing more and more. Eventually we realized he was having manic episodes. He got hospitalized and got medication, and he doesn't like the medication but he really needs it. Another time he stopped taking his meds, flew to Jerusalem on a whim because he thought he was going to get baptized, find God, or connect with Jesus or something. And we're Jewish!

—Josh, a sophomore describing his brother's manic episodes

I had all of the symptoms, until I got my bipolar under control. Shopping and crypto buying spree, betting on stuff like video games that racked up huge debt, really stupid investments, hooking up with everyone in sight, all stuff that I later learned were signs of mania. I just thought I was a fun person! These days I take medication, I honestly don't like it—a manic episode really feels incredible, like a cocaine rush that lasts a few weeks, but someone pointed out that like coke the negative consequences of both are pretty bad. I've got a solid support network now to help me see how damaging my manic episodes can be and to take my stupid meds.

—Lena, senior at a large private university

So What's Bipolar Disorder? Or Bipolar I Versus Bipolar II? Or Hypomanic Episodes? Or Cyclothymia?

Let's break this down. *Hypomania* is basically a lower-level mania, with at least three of those manic symptoms previously mentioned, lasting at least four days. *Bipolar disorder* is swinging between manias, and those depressive episodes that we also described earlier. All of these are very treatable with medications, and it's critical to take your medication even when you feel normal again; if you don't, the bipolar can worsen over the course of your lifetime with what's called "the kindling effect." It's also important to keep meeting with a therapist, who can help you find other coping strategies and also help you see when a manic episode may be starting, which is very hard to see from the inside.

Bipolar I includes swings between full mania and other moods, while *Bipolar II* is characterized as swinging between those milder "hypomanic" episodes and depression. *Cyclothymia* involves some hypomanic episodes over the years, but without depression. Remember though, this book is not diagnostic; it's about rough descriptions. These diagnostic nuances are really something to sort out with your provider rather than worrying too much about the specifics here, unless you're using the book to study for your psychopathology test.

How Do People Manage Manic and Bipolar Episodes?

More than many other disorders, bipolar disorder and mania need to be treated with mood-stabilizing medications. Especially when first diagnosed, someone requires a lot of check-ins with a prescriber, therapist, or support network, since many people recently diagnosed tend to be skeptical of medications, or often feel they are doing better and then stop. Mania itself feels so good that often people stop medications because they think they are feeling better, but it's the start of an episode.

What Is Psychosis?

Psychosis is a serious and significant "break from reality." Although psychosis is very extreme in its presentation and treatment and might bring about some fear, less than 0.3% of students have a psychotic disorder, so the likelihood that you will encounter it is rare.[5]

Psychosis can include hallucinations—seeing or hearing things like voices or spirits that do not exist in reality. There might be delusions—believing things that are not true like bizarre conspiracy theories (that often have the person at the center of them) or that they are being spied on. A person might experience "disordered thinking" with scattered ideas and thoughts coming rapidly and randomly, making nonsensical or bizarre statements.

Psychosis may be part of a diagnosable mental illness which is typically a more chronic condition. But it can also emerge temporarily from a sudden trigger, including severe stress, lack of sleep, and definitely substance use. Psychotic disorders are a group of serious illnesses that can make it hard for someone to think and perceive the world clearly and accurately, which in turn impairs judgment, communication, and behavior, and can become very dangerous when people have a major break from reality.

We want to emphasize, unlike other issues where people are aware of how strange their thoughts are and that causes more distress, with psychosis, people are more likely to fully believe them, and not even worry that their thinking is so bizarre. Sadly, it's almost always others who notice before the person themselves.

What Are Psychotic Disorders?

The most well-known psychotic disorder is *schizophrenia*—it's diagnosed when psychotic symptoms have lasted for more than six months. *Schizophreniform disorder* typically includes symptoms of schizophrenia, but for a shorter time, between one and six months. *Schizoaffective disorder* and *mood disorders with psychotic features* include overlapping mood and psychotic symptoms; however, in the latter, the psychosis only occurs in a mood episode.

What Are the Symptoms of a Psychotic Episode?

Hallucinations

A hallucination is a perception in our senses that seems real, but isn't. The most common hallucinations are auditory and visual, which means seeing and hearing things that are not really there.

Red Flags for You

☐ *Do you hear voices, maybe even telling you what to do, but when you look around no one is talking to you?*

☐ *Do you see things in your field of vision, or out of the corner of your eye, but then when you look around there is no one or nothing there?*

☐ *Do you ever have doubts about whether what you're seeing and hearing are real?*

Red Flags for Your Support Network

☐ *Does the person seem to be talking to themselves, or responding to unknown people?*

☐ *Do they appear to be looking at things that aren't there or you can't see?*

☐ *Are they describing things to you that literally aren't there?*

Delusions

A delusion is a false belief about external reality despite incontrovertible evidence to the contrary. It's a little different than anxious worries. Typically they are one of the following types. *Persecutory delusions* are when a person believes that someone or some group is planning to spy on them, get them, hurt them, control or even kill them. This might be worries that the CIA or FBI, or freemasons or illuminati, are out to get them, or in some people, demons or spirits. Then there are *grandiose delusions* when a person believes they have immense power, authority, or dominion over others, sometimes even magical powers. Maybe they think they have the ear of the university president or the ability to change things with the power of their mind. They might also think that others, including celebrities or politicians, are sending them hidden messages through social media that only they can understand.

Red Flags for You

☐ *Are you excessively worried about someone or some organization trying to hurt you or is spying on you?*

☐ *Is this getting in the way of you leaving your house, completing tasks, or in other ways that are disruptive to your daily life or wellbeing?*

☐ *Do you believe that you have some special powers or extra influence over others or life?*

☐ *Do you think that this puts you above others?*

☐ *Are you preoccupied with conspiracy theory content?*

Red Flags for Your Support Network

☐ *Does the person talk about people or groups that are spying on them, out to get them, or trying to control them?*

☐ *Do they have a massively inflated sense of power or what they are capable of, or talk about relationships with people that you know they don't know?*

continued

Confused and disturbed thoughts and behaviors

People with psychosis often have disturbed, rapidly changing thinking and disconnected, confused, and disjointed patterns of thinking that come out verbally. Outwardly that looks like rapid and nearly uninterruptible speech, bouncing between unrelated ideas. It may also look like an abrupt pause in conversation and activity. At times people with psychosis will copy other people's behavior, also as if mimicking them, or will stop and start smiling, making faces or crying when the situation is neither funny nor sad. While these are a reaction to what's going on in the person's brain, the person struggling often does not realize what's happening.

Red Flags for You

- ☐ *Although it can be difficult to distinguish between reality and psychosis, are you noticing that it is harder to concentrate?*
- ☐ *Do you hear voices of people telling you what to do, and in particular to do negative actions like hurt yourself or hurt other people?*
- ☐ *Do you see things or people out of the corner of your eye that aren't there?*
- ☐ *Do you believe people are out to get you or control you?*

Red Flags for Your Support Network

- ☐ *Does the person seem paranoid?*
- ☐ *Do they seem to be talking in a conversation when no one else is around?*

Decline in self-care or personal hygiene

Hygiene is one of the symptoms that are not frequently discussed when thinking about many mental health conditions. That's because it can be awkward to talk about, and people feel further stigmatized or embarrassed when asked about their hygiene habits, or it even drives others away from conversations. Nevertheless, indifference to daily hygiene tasks, like showering, brushing teeth, managing menstruation, doing laundry, or even simply brushing hair, is common with psychosis, as well as depression.

Red Flags for You

- ☐ *Have you stopped or reduced daily hygiene care such as showering and brushing your teeth?*

☐ *Have you been sleeping in the same sheets or wearing the same clothing without having washed them (more than the average college student)?*

☐ *Are people commenting or sending nonverbal cues about your personal appearance or body odor?*

☐ *This might be awkward but can indicate that your mental health is deteriorating.*

Red Flags for Your Support Network

☐ *Is the person not bathing, shaving, wearing deodorant, changing clothes, or brushing their teeth?*

☐ *Roommates are often the first to notice these signs, or parents on visiting weekends, especially if the person is isolating from others.*

What Happens If Someone Is Psychotic?

Generally, if someone is experiencing these psychotic symptoms, they'll be hospitalized and thoroughly evaluated, and typically leave school for a time to be medicated and stabilized. Sometimes it is a *brief psychotic disorder*, when students have a sudden, short period of psychotic behavior, often in response to a very stressful event, lack of sleep, or more likely, the use of certain drugs. In these circumstances, recovery is often quick, typically a few days or weeks. If the psychotic episode is triggered by drugs, it is termed *substance-induced psychotic disorder*. This is often caused by the use of, and sometimes withdrawal from, drugs or alcohol.

Although many drugs can cause psychosis, the most common on campuses include cannabis, psychedelics like psilocybin and LSD, and "club drugs" such as ketamine, ecstasy, and MDMA; even cocaine, and amphetamines in higher doses or when used for longer periods, can cause psychosis. Also, we are here to remind you that weed is not harmless and also is a common hallucinogen. The psychotic symptoms from drugs include visual hallucinations, disorientation, and paranoia. Although these types of psychotic experiences are very disturbing for everyone, sleep, food, rest, and the drug wearing off typically end the episode.

I remember hospitalizing a student who was having delusions that the school's public safety officers were spying on her through the keyholes in all of the rooms of her off-campus apartment, along with other bizarre worries. She went to the hospital and ended up discharged a day or so later after she'd gotten some rest (she'd been up for three nights doing a number of different drugs, including mari-juana, cocaine, benzodiazepines, Ritalin, and alcohol), and the effects of the drugs had worn off. I actually felt that she needed substance abuse treatment, but she returned for the rest of the semester, and two years later she took time off for substance misuse.

—**Chris, coauthor of this book**

How Is Psychosis Treated?

Often, schizophrenia and mood disorders with psychotic features require long-term medications and community mental health support and management, and some research indicates cognitive behavioral therapy can be helpful; talk therapy is much less helpful than medication.

> I don't know if this will be helpful for people reading your book, but I think the best way I can describe seeing my roommate have a psychotic episode was like talk-ing to someone on drugs. Like hallucinogens—acid or shrooms or something. Just making no sense, not connecting his mind to the real world, ranting about really weird ideas and conspiracies.
>
> —**Thomas, roommate of a student who had a psychotic episode**

> I remember a girl being sent over to the counseling center. We walked upstairs and behind me she was just talking about how she thought she had autism, and then that her pet bird has autism, and then kept talking about how she had created this new kind of math that only people and animals with autism could understand, and on and on with nonsense and jumping from idea to idea. We weren't even halfway up the stairs before I knew I was going to hospitalize her for psychosis.
>
> —**Hannah, therapist at a small Midwestern college**

In Conclusion

Mood disorders really are different than just moodiness, a bad day, or times of elation. At their worst, they can be deadly due to suicidal symptoms, or when it comes to bipolar disorder, they can present as impulsivity and an inability to judge risk. Psychosis, while rare, needs immediate attention because someone can pose a danger to themselves or others. We hope you now have a better sense from students and professionals of what the lived experience of these illnesses is really like, not just what we hear in pop culture or read in our textbooks.

Chapter 12

Behavioral Disorders

Borderline Personality Disorder, Self-Harm, Eating Disorders, and Addictions

Borderline personality disorder, self-harm, eating disorders, and substance misuse are themselves something of a grab bag of diagnoses, but all tend to involve behaviors with major consequences or side effects, and so we've put them together in this chapter. They are also some of the issues that have the most stigma and shame, and often they are the most misunderstood. We hope that this chapter can help you understand and manage these issues and behaviors, and get them under control, or at least more under control and manageable.

What Is Borderline Personality Disorder?

Borderline personality disorder (BPD) is a condition that impacts millions of people, and because of its nature, it also impacts the friends and families of those who are suffering from it. Although BPD is not something many have heard of, it is far more common than many other disorders. One study[1] showed the prevalence of BPD on college campuses as ranging from 0.5% to 32.1%, and a later study[2] found that 21.4% of the sample screened positive for BPD. An even more recent study[3] using an online survey of more than 12,000 students, found that compared to previous research, there was a significant increase in BPD symptoms for all sexes, with a particularly steep rise in female-identified students. The researchers also found that BPD symptoms significantly increased during the COVID-19 pandemic.

BPD typically affects five areas of functioning:

1. Struggle to regulate emotions
2. Experience volatile relationships
3. Behave in impulsive and self-destructive ways
4. Have significant distortions in thinking and perceiving
5. Struggle with having a consistent sense of self

As with all the diagnoses, many might recognize symptoms in themselves, and so it is important to get a formal expert diagnosis rather than trying to do this yourself. Nevertheless, if you experience some of these symptoms, you might want to seek a formal evaluation.

While many people have bad days, feeling low or irritable, for those with BPD, a bad mood makes it difficult to get almost anything done. A good mood is just the opposite; we call this *mood-dependent behavior.*

What Are the Symptoms of BPD?

Frantic efforts to avoid being abandoned, whether the threat is real or not

Red Flags for You

- [ ] *No one wants to be abandoned, especially by the people we care about or have just met. But people with BPD often present with a constant and overwhelming fear of abandonment. Do you wonder if you are "too much" or too needy?*
- [ ] *Do you worry constantly that your friends or romantic partner is going to ditch you?*
- [ ] *Do you want to constantly check if they still care about you or need the reassurance that you still matter to them?*

Red Flags for Your Support Network

- [ ] *Does the person seek reassurance, beg forgiveness, or people-please way more than necessary?*
- [ ] *Maybe they overtext partners or their friends or overshare information with everyone. Do they worry excessively about being excluded or left out?*
- [ ] *Do these constant needs for reassurance ever feel like they cross a line into what might feel manipulative?*
- [ ] *Do others say that the person is too dramatic, needy, or clingy?*

Intense and unstable relationships that swing between idealizing and villainizing others

Red Flags for You

☐ Do you fall hard for and idealize other people, whether sudden best friends or romantic partners, and get too invested too soon?

☐ Do these intense connections and infatuations happen frequently, only to end in heartbreak and anger, and the cycle begins again with another person?

Red Flags for Your Support Network

☐ Does the person wax glowingly about their latest romantic interest or best friend?

☐ Do they spend excessive amounts of time with the person and then seemingly turn on them quickly?

☐ Do they do it to you? Do their past and present relationships sound volatile?

☐ Do they seem to have a new best friend, new enemy or rival constantly?

A persistent lack of sense of self

Red Flags for You

☐ Do you frequently change life goals, your gender or sexual identity, or your interests like music and fashion, more than other students around you?

☐ Are those passions and decisions often similar to those of people you idealize?

This is beyond just doubts about internships and majors and the standard social swirl of college. It's more like going all in on one thing, and then switching, again and again.

Red Flags for Your Support Network

☐ Are they joining new groups and activities, talking excitedly about this being "the thing," and then switching suddenly to another, thinking that the new activity is the perfect match?

☐ You see them in one style one week, and then switching to a different fashion sense often based on others, and then switching again and again. Maybe they're

continued

an ardent supporter of one philosophical or political viewpoint and then rapidly switch and see the previous ones as totally wrong or bad.

Episodes of impulsive and potentially risky behaviors.

Red Flags for You

☐ *Do you engage in frequent unprotected or dangerous sexual behavior, often because you want connection, or even out of spite?*

☐ *Do you spend too much money shopping or gambling because of the thrill of the shopping or the high of the bet?*

☐ *Do you use drugs, less because of fitting in and more in order to change strong emotions?*

Red Flags for Your Support Network

☐ *Are you worried about this friend's choices about hookups and substances?*

☐ *Does it seem like there's a new bad decision every week?*

☐ *Does your friend use drugs when they are on their own, and seemingly because they appear to be self-medicating?*

Suicidal behavior and self-injury

Red Flags for You

☐ *Do you experience passive suicidal thoughts, imagining you'd be better off dead or not caring if an accident happened?*

☐ *Do you have the thought that suicide would end your problems?*

☐ *Have you ever made a suicide plan or acted, even partly, on suicidal thoughts?*

☐ *Do you have such intense emotions that cutting, scratching, or burning yourself makes you feel better?*

☐ *Or so numb that self-harm makes you feel more alive?*

Red Flags for Your Support Network

☐ *Does the person talk a lot about death or suicide?*

☐ *Do you notice scars or scratches, or are they covering arms and legs on hot days, or "accidentally" revealing them? Have you found razors, sharp objects, or bloody tissues?*

Large swings of emotions and moods

Red Flags for You

☐ *Do your emotions swing wildly and unpredictably, like an emotional roller coaster out of control?*

☐ *Do you feel guilty or ashamed over seemingly trivial matters?*

Red Flags for Your Support Network

☐ *Are you confused about your friend's unpredictable mood swings—are they happy one moment and then irritable, sad, or angry the next?*

☐ *Do you feel like you are "walking on eggshells" around this person, worried that you are going to set them off?*

Feeling empty, disconnected, or lonely a lot of the time

Red Flags for You

☐ *Do you often feel all alone even though you are surrounded by people, beyond the typical college homesickness?*

☐ *Do you feel perpetually misunderstood, like no one "gets" you at all?*

☐ *Do you feel that you don't belong anywhere?*

Red Flags for Your Support Network

☐ *Is this person hard to connect with?*

☐ *Do they complain about feeling disconnected or bored? Do you see growing pessimism or them making more negative comments?*

Excessive and intense anger, getting physical with people, destroying property, or being verbally cruel

Red Flags for You

☐ *Do you often feel that you are being taken advantage of or intentionally excluded?*

☐ *Does this make you want to lash out or get revenge or "teach someone a lesson"?*

☐ *Do you want to hurt others the way that you feel hurt?*

continued

Red Flags for Your Support Network

- [ ] *Do they often complain of being treated unfairly even for trivial seeming concerns?*
- [ ] *Do you worry about this person's lashing out physically or verbally in vengeful ways?*

Episodes of paranoia precipitated by stress, or feeling as if you are not real or the rest of the world does not feel real

Red Flags for You

- [ ] *Do you feel like people are conspiring against you?*
- [ ] *When you hear laughter, do you often assume people are laughing at you?*
- [ ] *Do have frequent times when you or the world doesn't feel "real"?*

Red Flags for Your Support Network

- [ ] *Does the person act abnormally suspicious of others, friends, peers, even adults, assuming bad intentions of others?*
- [ ] *Do they appear to space out when talking about painful memories?*

Other symptoms that are not in the Diagnostic and Statistical Manual of Mental Disorders (DSM) include a sense of loss of continuity of time, feeling constantly misunderstood, and significant self-hatred.

Red Flags for You

- [ ] *Do you feel that you have poor memory or disagree with others about remembering events?*
- [ ] *Do you feel enduring self-hatred?*

Red Flags for Your Support Network

- [ ] *Does this person remember things very differently than everyone else, maybe making you wonder if they're lying or gaslighting you or even themselves?*

For BPD, anger has been my biggest issue. I feel like yelling at my roommate; and when I look back, it was often for a small issue, but it didn't feel like that at the time.

—Maia, senior at a medium-sized private university

Finding an outlet is important. Poetry is really helpful for me. I can write my thoughts and rearrange them in a way that is beautiful. It also gives me a feeling that I can make something out of this pain. I also vent in my Notes app. Holding it in definitely results in a lot of destructive behavior. . . . And having one person in your life who you can trust, even if it's just a therapist, also helps.

—Priya, first-year student at a small liberal arts college

I like to do an ice dive when I'm overwhelmed with emotions. I fill a big bowl with cold water and ice cubes and dunk my face in it. I just do like three dives and it helps me feel more balanced.

—Winona, student at a small public university

I have permission from my daughter to hear about how she's doing from her therapist. It has been really helpful because I have a better idea of what to do. For example, the therapist said that I should stay with my daughter longer when she was having a breakdown to help her calm down and do a pros and cons list to make a decision about how to move forward, which was helpful advice. She also teaches my daughter DBT [dialectical behavioral therapy] skills which is helpful.

—Alice, mother of a student with BPD

I think the biggest thing that I've realized is that I can't be half of myself and give the best version of myself to my daughter or anyone else. It helps me also model to my child that it's important to take care of your needs. I would say, "I can't do xyz" for my self-care, but it is worth it and I deserve it. I also can't tell my daughter to do mindfulness and not make time to do it myself. It's helped, too, to connect with other parents of kids with BPD and feel not so alone on the roller coaster.

—Carol, mother of a student with BPD

How Is BPD Treated?

The most helpful treatment for BPD appears to be dialectical behavioral therapy (DBT) (Chapter 4). To recap, DBT teaches four main skill sets: mindfulness, emotion regulation, interpersonal effectiveness, and distress tolerance. Given that people with BPD struggle with staying present, regulating their emotions, relational turmoil, and tolerating distress, you can see why this would be the case.

What Is Nonsuicidal Self-Harm?

Self-harm is the behavior of intentionally injuring your own body. This can include cutting, burning, self-hitting, scratching, or punching a wall. The vast majority of self-injury actions are *not* with suicide in mind. That being said, people who self-harm are more likely to make suicide attempts and have other mental health issues.

The *DSM* says that self-harm is diagnosed when "in the last year, the individual has on five or more days, engaged in intentional self-inflicted damage to the surface of their body for purposes not socially sanctioned." "Socially sanctioned" would be activities like piercings and tattoos.

Most people who self-harm start in middle adolescence, and the second most frequent time is between 17 and 24, which means that the college years are a high-risk time for beginning self-injury, and definitely for potential relapse. In the largest review of all studies in self-injury in college,[4] the researchers estimated as many as 20% of college students engage in self-harm, with others indicating between 7% and 44%.[5]

Why Do People Self-Injure?

As you read this, you might be confused by the idea of self-harm, yet for many who self-harm, brain research shows that it has a calming effect,[6] explaining why it's so common.

Broadly speaking, there are three main reasons that students self-injure:

1. To help cope with intense emotions and intrusive thoughts. Some people self-harm because it blunts the impact and intensity of painful emotions. Self-injury works by releasing chemicals like cortisol, which regulate fight-or-flight response, lessening the impact of strong emotions, even if just temporarily.
2. To redirect emotions inward. Others may do so to punish or take their anger out on themselves. Still others who feel numb say they self-harm in order to feel anything but the numbness.
3. To communicate with others that they are in distress or want support. It is a common misconception that people who cut are "attention seeking." This occurs in fewer than 10% of cases, although it can be a way to communicate distress when nothing else seems to help.

Red Flags for You

- ☐ *Does it feel like your emotions are too much to bear?*
- ☐ *Do you feel so numb that you simply want to feel anything in order to feel alive?*
- ☐ *Do you ever feel that you deserve punishment?*
- ☐ *Do these thoughts come with the thought of hurting yourself?*
- ☐ *Does the thought of cutting yourself bring you some emotional relief?*

Red Flags for Your Support Network

- ☐ *Do you notice scars on the person?*
- ☐ *Have you seen razors and sharps around the room without a clear purpose?*
- ☐ *Have you found bloody tissues around, bloodstains on clothes, lots of bandages?*
- ☐ *Do they wear long sleeves or leggings even on very warm days?*
- ☐ *Do you ever wonder if they are "accidentally" revealing these for you to find?*

How Is Self-Harm Treated, and What Are Other Ways to Cope?

DBT and group therapy generally appear to be the most helpful for reducing self-harm.[7]

> I had a roommate freshman year who was a cutter. None of us knew for the whole first semester; she covered it really well. It was her boyfriend who told us he saw fresh cuts on her legs when they were hooking up. It was really hard to know what to do, but we went to the RA [resident advisor] who did a floorwide meeting on self-harm without calling her out specifically. That seemed like a helpful approach. I don't know what happened after that, but I think she got the help she needed.
> —**Lauren, sophomore at a large public university**

What Are Eating Disorders? And What Is Disordered Eating?

While eating disorders often begin in adolescence, it's during the college years that young people, especially young women, are at the highest risk. There's far less oversight of what you are eating and how much you are exercising, and far more social pressure around body image, than there was in high school.

According to the National Eating Disorders Association (NEDA), eating disorders typically begin between 18 and 21 years of age, and 10%–20% of women and 4%–10% of men in college suffer from an eating disorder, with rates for all genders on the rise.[8] However, these numbers are for full-blown eating disorders. Somewhere between 20% and 67% of your fellow students will exhibit "disordered eating," and unhealthy relationships to body image, exercise, and the like. Still, only 10% of women with eating disorders get help, and even fewer men do. In one study,[9] researchers recognized that while many students diet occasionally, 35% of regular dieters progressed to problematic dieting, and of those, nearly a quarter progressed to partial or full-on eating disorder diagnoses.

Eating disorders are not harmless; in fact, they have the highest mortality rate[10] of any mental illness. Five out of 1,000 people with anorexia, 1.7 of every 1,000 people with bulimia, and 3.3 people of 1,000 with other eating disorders will die from the eating disorder. The bottom line is that if you or a friend has an eating disorder, it can be deadly serious.

The eating options on college campuses, let alone food delivery apps, further complicate the problem. Often the freedom to eat or not eat whenever you want, along with a huge range of meal plans with no one looking over your shoulder, makes the college environment particularly dangerous for those already at risk. In high school, caregivers serve you a plate of food, but in college, you can literally have anything, everything, or nothing. Where Chelsie and Chris went, there was an ice cream station every night in the dining hall, not far from the salad bar, almost allowing anyone to choose their own eating issues.

Dr. Roberto Olivardia, an eating disorder specialist at Harvard Medical School, reminds us that if you're a little shy or socially anxious, you may find yourself avoiding the dining halls altogether. If you have executive function issues or take medication, it can be hard to remember to eat or get a regular routine around three healthy meals. Depression and anxiety can reduce your appetite or promote unhealthy or impulsive eating, even when you're not hungry. Adding stress to underlying mental health issues, along with the sense of a lack of control and not being monitored by parents, can push disordered eating into full-blown eating disorders.

It is important to note that there is a difference between an eating disorder and disordered eating. Disordered eating behaviors range from engaging in the latest fad diet every few months, including excluding certain food groups or calorie types, to behaviors like overexercising, misusing laxatives and stimulants such as nicotine and attention-deficit/hyperactivity disorder (ADHD) medications to suppress appetite, or eating things like hot sauce or drinking excessive water. None of these meet criteria for an eating disorder, but they are disordered eating behaviors, for which therapy can help.

What Is Binge Eating Disorder?

This is the most common eating disorder and describes compulsively overeating. It occurs when someone feels that they are unable to stop eating or have any control over the overeating.

The criteria include the following:

A. Eating a much larger amount of food than a typical person in a short amount of time. This excludes cultural feasts or eating for athletic training. The person also feels out of control and like they can't stop.

   The binges typically include at least three of the following:
   1. Eating much faster than you would normally
   2. Eating until you feel uncomfortably full
   3. Eating large amounts of food even when you are not particularly hungry
   4. Eating alone or hiding eating because of shame or embarrassment
   5. Feeling disgusted with yourself
B. The binges cause significant distress.
C. They occur at least once a week for at least three months.
D. The binges are not associated with purging or vomiting.

Red Flags for You

☐ Do you eat excessive amounts of food in short periods, even when not hungry?
☐ Do you feel overfull?
☐ Do you often feel disgusted, ashamed, or guilty about your eating?
☐ Do you eat alone or hide food and wrappers so that others won't see?

Red Flags for Your Support Network

☐ Does the person seem to eat alone, eat late at night, or you never see them eating?
☐ Do you find food missing from the fridge?
☐ Are there signs your roommate is hiding food or candy, like hiding wrappers in the trash?

What Is Bulimia?

This is the eating disorder when someone binge eats (above), but then engages in extreme behaviors to prevent weight gain.

The symptoms have to include the following:

A. Regular binges of food, often unhealthy foods.
B. Unhealthy or excessive behaviors to prevent weight gain like vomiting, using laxatives, diuretics, or drugs like stimulants; or long periods of food restriction, fasting, or excessive exercise
C. These cycles happen about once a week for three months.
D. Self-worth is excessively tied to body image.

Red Flags for You

☐ *Do you binging excessively, often high-calorie "junk food" over a short period of time?*
☐ *Do you beat yourself up and go to extremes to keep off the weight?*
☐ *Are you misusing medications, vomiting, or excessively exercising?*
☐ *Are you constantly worried about your weight, body shape, and appearance to the point it's hard to focus?*

Red Flags for Your Support Network

☐ *Is the person constantly commenting about being too fat or talking about calories?*
☐ *Do you notice signs of laxatives or other medications?*
☐ *Do they often eat a lot and later not at all, or exercise compulsively?*
☐ *Do they not eat with others?*
☐ *Do you hear or see signs of vomiting, including discolored or damaged teeth and gums, or spending excessive time in the bathroom after eating?*
☐ *Does their weight or body shape fluctuate significantly?*
☐ *Often coaches, teammates, and people at the gym are the first to notice eating disorders.*

What Is Anorexia?

Anorexia is an eating disorder where the person has an abnormally low body weight, an intense fear of gaining weight, and an extremely distorted sense of how they look. They feel overweight no matter the evidence from others, including doctors. People with anorexia place a high value on controlling their weight and shape, often going to such extreme efforts to keep their weight so low that it interferes with functioning and becomes dangerous.

Anorexia includes the following:

1. Eating far fewer calories than needed, leading to a significantly, often dangerously low body weight.
2. An intense fear or intrusive fear of gaining weight, despite being underweight by all objective measures.
3. A misperception of body weight or shape and extreme connection between weight and self-concept. Frequent denial and self-denial about the seriousness of the low body weight or health considerations.

Although the *DSM* does not include the physical and psychological consequences of anorexia in the diagnostic criteria, many of the symptoms can significantly impact college life.

Physical symptoms

Many of these symptoms would impact academic and social life on campus.

- Dangerously low red blood cell counts and potassium levels
- Fatigue
- Insomnia
- Dizziness or fainting
- Hair that thins, breaks, or falls out
- Absence of menstruation
- Constipation and abdominal pain
- Irregular heartbeat

Behavioral symptoms

Can include attempts to lose weight by the following, and again you can see how some of these could have a significant impact on your college experience:

continued

- Severely restricting food intake through dieting or fasting
- Exercising excessively
- Binging and self-induced vomiting to get rid of the recently eaten food. Although students often believe that others are not aware, it is typically the case that they are.
- A preoccupation with food, and sometimes includes cooking elaborate meals, or making calorie-rich food for others but not eating the food themselves
- Frequently skipping meals or refusing to eat, which can make it hard to socialize
- Adopting rigid eating rituals, such as spitting food out after chewing or cutting up food into small pieces and moving the food around on the plate
- Lying about the amount of food that has been eaten
- Frequently checking mirrors or windows to check for observable weight gain
- A reduced interest in sex or romantic relationships

Emotional symptoms

Are often the manifestation of a starving brain and can include the following:

- Covering up in layers of clothing in order to avoid other people commenting on weight
- A lack of emotional experience, a flatness of mood
- Social withdrawal
- Feeling irritable and easily set off by the seemingly smallest provocation
- Insomnia, and then anxiety about the insomnia
- Difficulty focusing

Red Flags for You

☐ *Do you eat very small amounts of food, if at all?*
☐ *Are you constantly worried about your weight and appearance?*
☐ *Do you obsess about calories, worry that you are going to become fat, even as others say you are too thin?*
☐ *Do you constantly look in mirrors or windows, or weigh yourself to see if there is any sign of weight gain?*

Is your hair falling out, or is short fuzzy hair growing on your body? Do you feel dizzy and weak or notice heart palpitations? Do you buy others calorie-rich food and feel some relief that they are putting on weight and that you are not?

Red Flags for Your Support Network

☐ *Does the person eat alone, or not at all, or not go to the dining hall with you?*

□ *Do they push around food on their plate to hide how much they are eating?*

□ *Do they seem stressed or avoidant about eating and mealtimes, constantly commenting on calories?*

□ *Are they excessively thin, developing more hair on their arms or face, or showing gaunt facial features?*

□ *Do they eat only things like celery or hot sauce and spend too many hours exercising?*

How Are Eating Disorders Best Treated?

Typically eating disorders require specialist treatment, sometimes even hospitalization. A treatment team typically includes an eating disorder therapist, nutritionist, or registered dietician and psychiatrist.

Substance Misuse—When Does It Go From a Party to a Problem?

The difference between substance use and misuse can be difficult to differentiate. This is because in the college years, a lot of students overindulge. There are specific signs to look out for to distinguish between social excess and concerning.

DSM Symptoms of Substance Misuse

Taking a substance in a larger amount or over a longer period than intended.

Red Flags for You

□ *Maybe you only planned to have four drinks and next thing you knew you were waking up with little memory. You planned to go out partying only a few nights, but it turned into more. Thinking that the amount of drugs or alcohol will last longer than it actually does. Telling yourself you'll sell a little and keep the rest, then using more than intended. Being the last one up still imbibing.*

continued

Red Flags for Your Support Network

☐ *Is the person consuming a lot rapidly, without slowing down?*
☐ *Using more, or more often than they said they would or used to?*
☐ *Are they doing a lot more, and later than the rest of the social group?*
☐ *Do you suspect they are pregaming on their own, or still using after most others have called it a night?*

Persistent desire or unsuccessful efforts to cut down or control substance use

Red Flags for You

☐ *Do you keep thinking you'll use/drink less and then don't?*
☐ *Do you tell yourself you won't use certain days/times and then do?*

Red Flags for Your Support Network

☐ *Are there broken promises or agreements to themself and others about how much or how often they'll use?*

Significant time obtaining, using, recovering from effects

Red Flags for You

☐ *Are you driving long distances or spending lots of time just getting drugs or pursuing the behavior?*
☐ *Going on longer benders and missing out on things?*
☐ *Spending time missing things because you are recovering from hangovers or dealing with withdrawal?*

Red Flags for Your Support Network

☐ *Are they not showing up for things due to using, buying, or recovering?*

Strong desires and craving

Red Flags for You

☐ *Do you feel a lot like you "really need" a drink or drug or behavior?*
☐ *Is it making it hard to focus on school or other things?*

☐ *Do you not feel like yourself unless you are indulging at least somewhat?*

Red Flags for Your Support Network

☐ *Are they frequently saying they need a drink/hit, and so on?*

☐ *Are they not acting or looking normal when they don't have access to the substance?*

☐ *Do they look or act "uncomfortable in their own skin" without the substance?*

☐ *Do they talk way too much about their plans or how much they want or need a drink or drug, etc?*

Failure to fulfill major role obligations at work, school, or home due to using

Red Flags for You

☐ *Do you sleep through work or school?*

☐ *Missing jobs, classes and appointments?*

☐ *Have you gotten so intoxicated you forgot social obligations?*

Red Flags for Your Support Network

☐ *Are they not getting things done, not showing up for friends, work, and school?*

Continued use despite persistent social or interpersonal problems caused or exacerbated by substance abuse

Red Flags for You

☐ *Are you still pursuing the substance or behavior despite ultimatums from friends and partners that they'll leave or break up with you?*

☐ *Are your parents or caregivers upset with your level of use?*

☐ *Are you spending too much of your money that you need for basic living expenses?*

Red Flags for Your Support Network

☐ *Are you noticing personality and behavior changes when they're using (angry, aggressive, sad, mean) or when in withdrawal?*

☐ *Do you see unpredictable behavior, mood swings, and personality changes, even when apparently sober?*

☐ *Are they breaking agreements?*

☐ *Are they asking for money and/or running out of money quickly?*

continued

Missing important social, occupational, or recreational activities because of substance abuse

Red Flags for You

☐ *Are you missing team practices, club and Greek activities and commitments?*
☐ *Not showing up to meetings for graduate school, career or study abroad?*
☐ *Behind on deadlines?*

Red Flags for Your Support Network:

☐ *Are they missing classes, study sessions, social events, extracurricular activities, or sports?*

Recurrent use in situations where it's physically dangerous

Red Flags for You

☐ *Have you had accidents or near accidents and injuries?*
☐ *Getting into dangerous activities like climbing or jumping from heights, break-ins, and so forth?*
☐ *Going to dangerous neighborhoods, getting into high risk situations?*
☐ *Have you been in legal or disciplinary trouble?*

Red Flags for Your Support Network

☐ *Are they still using often even after negative experiences like being injured, assaulted, robbed, or hospitalized?*
☐ *Are they risking disciplinary and legal consequences?*

Continued use despite persistent/recurrent physical or psychological problems that are likely caused or worsened by use.

Red Flags for You

☐ *Are the substances or lack of them increasing anxiety, depression, or other symptoms?*
☐ *Are you getting sick regularly but still using?*

Red Flags for Your Support Network

☐ *Are they continuing to use even when it worsens mood and depression, leads to more anxiety, worsens focus, in addition to possibly having physical issues and other side effects?*

Increased tolerance

Red Flags for You

☐ *Do you need a lot more to feel high or intoxicated?*
☐ *Are you taking "tolerance breaks?"*
☐ *Does it take much more than your friends to get the right buzz?*

Red Flags for Your Support Network

☐ *Do they need a lot more than they used to get high or feel what they used to?*
☐ *Are they using higher amounts more often?*
☐ *Are they using a lot and not appearing to feel the effects?*
☐ *Are they sneaking drinks, doses, pills, and bumps?*
☐ *Did they used to drink/use the same amount as their friend group, and now do much more?*

Withdrawal symptoms

Red Flags for You

☐ *Are you noticing physical or psychological differences and effects on days you're not using?*
☐ *Feeling sick, shaky, nauseous, headaches, hot and cold flashes, and others (depending on the substance), goosebumps, flu-like symptoms?*
☐ *Are you more depressed and anxious, irritable and unfocused when you're not using regularly?*

Red Flags for Your Support Network

☐ *Do you notice them missing things from being sick?*
☐ *Reporting physical symptoms like nausea, shakes, headaches, hot and cold flashes, and others (depending on the substance), goosebumps, flu-like symptoms?*

continued

☐ *Do you see psychological symptoms like anxiety, depression, irritability, difficulty focusing, and others when they aren't using?*

Irritability, restlessness

Red Flags for You

☐ *Are little things bothering you more than in the past?*
☐ *Less patience for people around you?*
☐ *Everyone and everything annoying you or feeling boring?*

Red Flags for Your Support Network

☐ *Do you notice they are grumpier, shorter tempered, more irritable than in the past?*
☐ *Are they struggling to stay on task?*

All of these are really hard to measure and quantify. Students who are high after smoking might forget where to meet friends, or they may be too hungover to get to the library. But it's when you lose those friendships, grades begin to suffer, your coach confronts you about your performance, your physical health is impacted, you black out, and these begin to happen regularly and you keep using, that it's a red flag that the substance is the problem.

Another concern is the development of tolerance, which means that you need to use a lot more of the substance than you did before to get the same sort of effect. When you begin using instead of fulfilling your basic social and academic responsibilities, this is when it becomes an issue.

There's a real chicken-and-egg problem when it comes to both understanding and treating substance use disorder. For example, many believe that "self-medicating" anxiety, trauma, depression, or other mental health issues is behind substance use, and if the mental health condition is treated, that the substance use will improve. Others feel like the substance use issue needs to be addressed first before the mental health issues can clear up. It can be either/or, and it is also possible that the substance use causes the mental health condition.

One of the things I look for is a very high tolerance off the bat. If they are drinking or using way more than their friends, whether they are getting more inebriated or not, that to me is often a red flag. Or, if they are getting more inebriated more often than the rest of the friend group, that's another flag.

—Jason, substance misuse educator at a large private university

There are other addictive behaviors that I think are important to recognize, and those are gambling and porn. With the legalization of sports betting, I've seen a lot of young folks, particularly guys, get in way over their heads in terms of gambling, racking up huge debt in ways that are not unlike substance abuse addiction, then hiding it or trying to gamble their way out. . . . Likewise, a lot of young men I work with are very unhappy with their relationship to pornography, which can bring up a lot of shame. Not everyone agrees that these are full-blown addictions, but many people agree that they are behaviors that can lead to big problems but also that can be treated.

—Mike, social worker and substance misuse evaluator

Yes, my friends drank, did coke, and all of that as well. It was part of the group I was in, and the atmosphere of the party school I went to. But I was often doing a shot or two in my room before meeting up with friends, an extra bump or two in the bathroom my sisters didn't know about, and some nights was still drinking and blowing lines even after everyone else was asleep. If you're doing any of those things, I'd say that's a sign of a problem.

—Claudia, recent college graduate of a large private southern university

I went to rehab and back to school, and relapsed and repeated the cycle a few times before it really stuck for me. The substance-free housing was not really my social scene, and living on my own, though isolating, was the least bad option for me. Finding the campus 12-step meetings was a lifesaver. I had students and staff who were sober who I could see around campus as little reminders. Over time I also shifted more of my social life to sober community in the town I was in school. There was a worker in the dining hall from one of my meetings, and seeing her was always reassuring. But overall, those last few years of school were not the typical college experience in that way, but at least I'm alive and sober.

—Rachel, junior at a large public university

What I noticed about a lot of young people I've seen successfully get sober over the years is that they found some meaning in their lives. It used to be that people said you had to find God or religion to get sober. But now I believe it can be anything meaningful. Maybe that is religion for some people, but maybe getting really into exercise or yoga, hiking and the outdoors, art or writing, or a meaningful job, or helping others in some way. . . . Once they found that, they were able to stay sober in the long run. I actually now think that's true not just for addiction, but a lot of issues.

—Chris, coauthor of this book

What else I want to emphasize is there is no rush. The more time you have sober, the more likely you are to stay sober when you get back to college, and then of course hopefully finding healthy living. The longer you are sober in treatment, or a halfway or sober living place, you also can look back with some good memories and have a track record of sobriety not being so bad and remember—'Oh, I can have fun sober, I can make friends sober, I can laugh my ass off sober'—then sobriety seems like a reasonable option, and you don't need the substances to feel good, or happy, or have fun.

—Kris Kampf, chemical dependency counselor

When we get together with friends, our brains release dopamine when we enjoy each other's company. That makes us want to do more of that. But when we smoke or drink together, we get the release, but jacking it up from the substance. So eventually hanging out isn't as fun anymore because there's a new set point. Over time, for some of us, is that consciously or unconsciously, we associate smoking with positive feelings and start to isolate and just use as the friendships fall away and friends and family begin to worry. Viewing alcohol as a way to manage anxiety or stress increases the risk of later dependence.

—Substance misuse educator in Massachusetts

In Conclusion

Folks find some mental health issues are easier to empathize with, while others are more difficult. BPD, self-harm, addiction, and eating disorders are at times perceived by others as willful, or like the person in question is doing the behaviors on purpose. We don't always know what is causing them, but we know that many people who struggle with these wish they could stop, and some struggle for months or years without relapsing back. Treatment is often time intensive, with intensive outpatient groups or hospitalizations to stabilize people until they are able to abstain or significantly reduce the behaviors. We hope that you or whoever you care about can get the best help that you need as soon as you can, and that you can move in a positive trajectory as quickly as possible.

Conclusion

"To be yourself in a world that is constantly trying to make you something else is the greatest accomplishment."

—Ralph Waldo Emerson

There is some idea out there that the college experience is supposed to look
one way. But there is no "one way" or "right way." Maybe you've heard
some of those eye-roll-inducing comments like "These are gonna be the best
four years of your life!" or "Everything you do right now is key because it will
set the tone for the rest of your life!"

Maybe yes, but maybe no.

So don't pay much attention to those sentiments if they don't resonate for
you. College, while it is a major milestone and achievement in one's life, it is,
at the end of the day, just another life experience. No added pressure needed.
Maybe you will realize what your purpose is or make the best friends you've
ever had. But maybe you won't, and your experience is *your* experience. And
if you have struggles with your mental health or experience stress for the first
time now, college can be a time when you realize that your self-care is more
under your control than you imagined, and certainly more than it has ever
been. (As a family member or friend, a loved one's challenges may also be
a chance to understand their struggle and learn how to be a support for the
people you care about in the way that they need.)

Especially if you have to put more effort into managing your mental health,
your college experience might just look and feel different from others, for
all or for part of your time. But sometimes we just want to feel "normal."
It's okay to grieve the fact that you're not having the experience that you
wanted to have, or maybe the one that you expected to have based on ideas
you got from high school, movies and TV, or some adults who shared their
own experiences. And it's okay to feel upset if you look around and your
experience seems to be lacking compared to those around you. So tend to
your heart first, and give yourself grace and space for whatever comes up
there.

It's easy to feel like you're not measuring up. The good news is that life
almost always works itself out. This is a secret that the pressures of society or

family don't make clear. This doesn't mean that you sit back passively when everything is going up in flames and just hope for the best, but if you feel like you've made a wrong turn, you can always reroute your life. It might take a little longer to get where you wanted to go, but you can absolutely still make it. The idea of "failure" is all a matter of perspective, and fortunately, you are in charge of how you choose to view things. You can see fire as something that is going to burn your house down or the energy necessary to cook your food. If you have to take a semester off to focus on your mental health, maybe that time away from college will help you realize what you want to do after graduation. Or if you have to drop a class because you got too far behind during a depressive episode, maybe the extra time that you have in your week will give you the space for some extra self-care that will revive you.

We know that these ideas are easier written about and easier said than done. Your own authors have been there. One of them took a year off of her studies because her mental health was in a dire state. Another took two years. It felt like too much, and it led to the question: "Why can't I just get through this?" But that time off allowed us the space to focus on healing and activities that brought us joy, outside of being productive or career focused, or even too focused on social stuff. And when we returned, we were in a much better place to be present in our experience, and we'd definitely say it all worked out in the end. We are writing this book, after all!

While this book couldn't possibly address everything about college mental health, we hope that it gives you some helpful information to get you through this time and gets you to the right resources so you are adequately supported. We also hope that you see yourself reflected in these pages. In some ways, we see this book as more than a book—we see it as a project, and we want to keep building on it. If you have stories, feedback, advice, or thoughts, don't hesitate to reach out to any of us. We're easily Googleable, and we welcome your thoughts if they can help us be better at our work with helping others.

We know that the college experience is filled with highs and lows, and we wish you balance on your journey to managing your mental health and all of the demands of the college experience. It certainly isn't easy, so don't forget to applaud yourself for still trying even when it gets tough.

Part of being an adult is managing your mental health. This is a lifelong practice beyond the specific circumstances of this moment and the context of college. College is not just the time to work toward your goals, passions, and purpose—it is also the time to create an emotionally nourishing foundation for the rest of your life. How you learn to care for yourself now matters going forward, and even if you feel behind, you may well come out ahead, having been through some of your biggest challenges when you were young. Maybe one day you'll share your wisdom with others.

We're rooting for you!

References

Introduction

1 Centers for Disease Control and Prevention. (n.d.). Suicide: Facts at a glance. Retrieved June 18, 2024, from https://www.cdc.gov/facts/index.html
2 National Education Association. (2023). *The mental health crisis on college campuses*. National Education Association. https://www.nea.org/nea-today/all-news-articles/mental-health-crisis-college-campuses
3 Jed Foundation. (n.d.). *Mental health and suicide statistics*. Retrieved June 18, 2024, from https://jedfoundation.org/mental-health-and-suicide-statistics/
4 National Alliance on Mental Illness. (n.d.). *Mental health conditions*. Retrieved June 18, 2024, from https://www.nami.org/about-mental-illness/mental-health-conditions/#:~:text=1%20in%2020%20U.S.%20adults,and%2075%25%20by%20age%2024
5 National Alliance on Mental Illness. (2012, December 19). *College survey: 50 percent of college students with mental health problems who withdraw from school because of mental health issues never access college mental health services*. Retrieved June 18, 2024, from https://www.nami.org/press-releases/college-survey-50-percent-of-college-students-with-mental-health-problems-who-withdraw-from-school-because-of-mental-health-issues-never-access-college-mental-health-services/#:~:text=ARLINGTON%2C%20VA%2C%20Dec.,on%20Mental%20Illness%20(NAMI).
6 Ballard Brief. (n.d.). *High suicide rates among young adults in the United States*. Retrieved June 18, 2024, from https://ballardbrief.byu.edu/issue-briefs/high-suicide-rates-among-young-adults-in-the-united-states
7 Jed Foundation. (n.d.). *Mental health and suicide statistics*. Retrieved June 18, 2024, from https://jedfoundation.org/mental-health-and-suicide-statistics/
8 Healthy Minds Network. (n.d.). *Healthy Minds Network*. Retrieved June 18, 2024, from https://healthymindsnetwork.org/hms/

Chapter 1

1 Bryn Mawr Access Services. (n.d.). Differences between idea IEPS, 504 plans, and college accommodations. Bryn Mawr College. https://www.brynmawr.edu/inside/offices-services/access-services/information-students/differences-between-idea-ieps-504-plans-college-accommodations

Chapter 3

1 American College Health Association. (2024). *American College Health Association–National College Health Assessment III: Undergraduate Student Reference Group Data Report Fall 2023*. Silver Spring, MD: American College Health Association.

2 Substance Abuse and Mental Health Services Administration. (2022). Key substance use and mental health indicators in the United States: Results from the 2021 National Survey on Drug Use and Health (HHS Publication No. PEP22-07-01-005, NSDUH Series H-57). Center for Behavioral Health Statistics and Quality, Substance Abuse and Mental Health Services Administration. https://www.samhsa.gov/data/report/2021-nsduh-annual-national-report

Chapter 4

1 Beck, A. T. (1976). *Cognitive therapy and the emotional disorders.* Madison, CT: International Universities Press.
2 Linehan, M. M. (1993). *Skills training manual for treating borderline personality disorder.* New York: Guilford Press.
3 Linehan, M. M. (1993). *Cognitive-behavioral treatment of borderline personality disorder.* Guilford Press.
4 Gillespie, C., Murphy, M., Kells, M., & Flynn, D. (2022). Individuals who report having benefitted from dialectical behaviour therapy (DBT): A qualitative exploration of processes and experiences at long-term follow-up. *Borderline Personality Disorder and Emotion Dysregulation, 9*(1), 8. https://doi.org/10.1186/s40479-022-00179-9
5 Cuddy, A. J. C., Wilmuth, C. A., & Yap, A. J. (2015). Power posing: Brief nonverbal displays affect neuroendocrine levels and risk tolerance. *Psychological Science, 21*(10), 1363–1368. https://doi.org/10.1177/0956797614553946

Chapter 5

1 Luo, Q., Zhang, P., Liu, Y., Ma, X., & Jennings, G. (2022). Intervention of physical activity for university students with anxiety and depression during the COVID-19 pandemic prevention and control period: A systematic review and meta-analysis. *International Journal of Environmental Research and Public Health, 19*(22), 15338. DOI: 10.3390/ijerph192215338. PMID: 36430056; PMCID: PMC9692258
2 Singh, B., Olds, T., Curtis, R., Dumuid D., Virgara R., Watson A., Szeto K., O'Connor E., Ferguson T., Eglitis E., Miatke A., Simpson, C. E., Maher, C. (2023). Effectiveness of physical activity interventions for improving depression, anxiety, and distress: An overview of systematic reviews. *British Journal of Sports Medicine, 57*, 1203–1209.
3 Morris, M. R., Hoeflich, C. C., Nutley, S., Ellingrod, V. L., Riba, M. B., and Striley, C. W. (2021). Use of psychiatric medication by college students: A decade of data. *Pharmacotherapy, 41*, 350–358. https://doi.org/10.1002/phar.2513
4 Marconi A. M., Myers U. S., Hanson B., Nolan S., Sarrouf E. B. (2023). Psychiatric medication prescriptions increasing for college students above and beyond the COVID-19 pandemic. *Scientific Reports, 13*(1), 19063. doi: 10.1038/s41598-023-46303-9. PMID: 37925588; PMCID: PMC10625532
5 Baker, E. A., & Miracle, T. L. (2022). College prescription drug study key findings report. Columbus: College of Pharmacy, The Ohio State University.
6 Almohammed, O. A., Alsalem, A. A., Almangour, A. A., Alotaibi, L. H., Al Yami, M. S., Lai, L. (2022). Antidepressants and health-related quality of life (HRQoL) for patients with depression: Analysis of the medical expenditure panel survey from the United States. *PLoS ONE, 17*(4), e0265928. https://doi.org/10.1371/journal.pone.0265928

7 Choi, C., Johnson, D. E., Chen-Li, D., & Rosenblat, J. (2024). Mechanisms of psilocybin on the treatment of posttraumatic stress disorder. *Journal of Psychopharmacology.*

8 Mithoefer, M. C., Designee, S., Doblin, R., Emerson, A., Mithoefer, A., Jerome, L., Ruse, J., Doblin, R., Gibson, E., Ot'alora, M., & Sola, E. (2017, August 22). A manual for MDMA-assisted psychotherapy in the treatment of posttraumatic stress disorder. Multidisciplinary Association for Psychedelic Studies. https://maps.org/wp-content/uploads/2022/05/MDMA-Assisted-Psychotherapy-Treatment-Manual-V8.1-22AUG2017.pdf

9 Schulenberg J. E., Johnston L. D., O'Malley, P. M., Bachman, J. G., Miech, R. A., Patrick, M. E. (2018). Monitoring the Future: National Survey Results on Drug Use, 1975–2017: Volume II, College Students and Adults Ages 19–55. National Institute of Drug Abuse.

Chapter 6

1 American College Health Association. 2024. American College Health Association–National College Health Assessment III: Reference Group Executive Summary Fall 2023. Silver Spring, MD: American College Health Association.

2 Droit-Volet, S., & Meck, W. H. (2007). How emotions colour our time perception. *Trends in Cognitive Science, 11,* 504–513. DOI: 10.1016/j.tics.2007.09.008

3 Center for Mindful Self-Compassion. (n.d.). Exercise 2: Self-compassion break. Retrieved June 23, 2024, from https://self-compassion.org/exercises/exercise-2-self-compassion-break/

Chapter 7

1 Norcross, J. C., Krebs, P. M., & Prochaska, J. O. (2011). Stages of change. *Journal of clinical psychology, 67*(2), 143–154. https://doi.org/10.1002/jclp.20758

2 Prochaska, J. O., & DiClemente, C. C. (1983). Stages and processes of self-change of smoking: Toward an integrative model of change. *Journal of Consulting and Clinical Psychology, 51*(3), 390–395. DOI: 10.1037/0022-006X.51.3.390

Chapter 8

1 Cage, E., & Howes, J. (2020). Dropping out and moving on: A qualitative study of autistic people's experiences of university. *Autism, 24*(7), 1664–1675. 10.1177/1362361320918750

2 Sedgwick, J. A. (2018). University students with attention deficit hyperactivity disorder (ADHD): A literature review. *Iranian Journal of Psychological Medicine, 35,* 221–235. 10.1017/ipm.2017.20.

3 Rajbhandari-Thapa, J., Chiang, K., Lee, M. C., Treankler, A., Padilla, H., Vall, E. A., & Fedrick, M. (2023). Depression and anxiety among college students at Historically Black and Predominantly White universities during the COVID-19 pandemic: A cross-sectional study. *Journal of American College Health, 24,* 1–8. DOI: 10.1080/07448481.2023.2230297. Epub ahead of print. PMID: 37,487,205.

4 Kreniske, P., Mellins, C. A., Shea, E., Walsh, K., Wall, M., Santelli, J. S., Reardon, L., Khan, S., Hwei, T., & Hirsch, J. S. (2023). Associations between low-household income and first-generation status with college student belonging, mental health, and well-being. *Emerging Adulthood, 11*(3), 710–720. https://doi.org/10.1177/21676968221124649

5 Gross, E. B., Kattari, S. K., Wilcox, R., Ernst, S., Steel, M., & Parrish, D. (2022). Intricate realities: Mental health among trans, nonbinary, and gender diverse college students. *Youth, 2*(4), 733–745. https://doi.org/10.3390/youth2040052

6 Minotti, B. J., Ingram, K. M., Forber-Pratt, A. J., & Espelage, D. L. (2021). Disability community and mental health among college students with physical disabilities. *Rehabilitation Psychology, 66*(2), 192–201. https://doi.org/10.1037/rep0000377

7 Park, E. Y., Oliver, T. R., Peppard, P. E., & Malecki, K. C. (2023). Sense of community and mental health: A cross-sectional analysis from a household survey in Wisconsin. *Family Medicine and Community Health, 11*(2), e001971. doi: 10.1136/fmch-2022-001971. PMID: 37,399,294; PMCID: PMC10314672.

8 Lee, R. M., Draper, M., & Lee, S. (2001). Social connectedness, dysfunctional interpersonal behaviors, and psychological distress: Testing a mediator model. *Journal of Counseling Psychology. 48*(3), 310–318.

9 Seppala, E. Connectedness and health: The science of social connection. The Center for Compassion and Altruism Research and Education, Stanford University. May 8, 2014. Accessed March 21, 2023. http://ccare.stanford.edu/uncategorized/connectedness-health-the-science-of-social-connection-infographic

10 Collins, P. H., & Bilge, S. (2020). *Intersectionality* (2nd ed.). Cambridge: Polity Press.

11 Noetel, M., Sanders, T., Gallardo-Gómez, D., Taylor, P., del Pozo Cruz, B., van den Hoek, D., Mahoney, J., Spathis, J., Moresi, M., Pagano, R., Vasconcellos, R., Arnott, H., Varley, B., Parker, P., Biddle, P., Lonsdal, C. (2024). Effect of exercise for depression: Systematic review and network meta-analysis of randomised controlled trials *BMJ,* 384, e075847. doi:10.1136/bmj-2023-075847

12 Eby, L. T., Allen, T. D., Evans, S. C., Ng, T., & Dubois, D. (2008). Does mentoring matter? A multidisciplinary meta-analysis comparing mentored and non-mentored individuals. *Journal of Vocational Behavior, 72*(2), 254–267. https://doi.org/10.1016/j.jvb.2007.04.005

13 Smith, D. G., & Schonfeld, N. B. (2000). The benefits of diversity: What the research tells us. *About Campus, 5*(5), 16–23. https://doi.org/10.1177/108648220000500505

14 Peteet, B. J., Montgomery, L., & Weekes, J. C. (2015). Predictors of imposter phenomenon among talented ethnic minority undergraduate students. *The Journal of Negro Education, 84*(2), 175–186. https://doi.org/10.7709/jnegroeducation.84.2.0175

15 Jones, K., and Okun, T. (2001). *White supremacy culture.*

Chapter 9

1 American Psychiatric Association. (2013). *Diagnostic and statistical manual of mental disorders* (5th ed., Text Revision). Washington, DC: American Psychiatric Association.

2 Clouder, L., Karakus, M., Cinotti, A., Ferreyra, M., Fierros, G., & Rojo, P. (2020). Neurodiversity in higher education: A narrative synthesis. *Higher Education, 80,* 757–778. https://doi.org/10.1007/s10734-020-00513-6

3 Mowlem, F., Agnew-Blais, J., Taylor, E., & Asherson, P. (2019). Do different factors influence whether girls versus boys meet ADHD diagnostic criteria? Sex differences among children with high ADHD symptoms. *Psychiatry Research, 272,* 765–773. https://doi.org/10.1016/j.psychres.2018.12.128

4 Hotez, E., Rosenau, K. A., Fernandes, P., Eagan, K., Shea, L., & Kuo, A. A. (2022). A national cross-sectional study of the characteristics, strengths, and challenges of college students with attention deficit hyperactivity disorder. *Cureus, 14*(1), e21520. https://doi.org/10.7759/cureus.21520

5 Heiligenstein, E., Guenther, G., Levy, A., Savino, F., & Fulwiler, J. (1999). Psychological and academic functioning in college students with attention deficit hyperactivity disorder. *Journal of American College Health, 47*(4), 181–185, DOI: 10.1080/07448489909595644

6 Mark, G., Iqbal, S., Czerwinski, M., Johns, P., & Sano, A. (2016). Neurotics Can't Focus: An in situ Study of Online Multitasking in the Workplace. 1739–1744. 10.1145/2858036.2858202.

7 McSpadden, K. (2015, May 14). *Science: You now have a shorter attention span than a goldfish.* Time. https://time.com/3858309/attention-spans-goldfish/

8 Supekar, K., de los Angeles, C., Ryali, S., Cao, K., Ma, T., & Menon, V. (2022). Deep learning identifies robust gender differences in functional brain organization and their dissociable links to clinical symptoms in autism. *The British Journal of Psychiatry, 220*(4), 202–209. doi:10.1192/bjp.2022.13

9 Stobbe, M. (2023, February 20). *Autism now more common among black, Hispanic kids in US.* AP News. https://apnews.com/article/how-common-is-autism-e38179682e2759b0aff9c017bf7ebf61

10 Jadav, N., & Bal, V. H. (2022). Associations between co-occurring conditions and age of autism diagnosis: Implications for mental health training and adult autism research. *Autism Research, 15*(11), 2112–2125. https://doi.org/10.1002/aur.2808

11 Shattuck, P. T., Narendorf, S. C., Cooper, B., Sterzing, P. R., Wagner, M., & Taylor, J. L. (2012). Postsecondary education and employment among youth with an autism spectrum disorder. *Pediatrics, 129*(6), 1042–1049. https://doi.org/10.1542/peds.2011-2864

12 Pinder-Amaker S. (2014). Identifying the unmet needs of college students on the autism spectrum. *Harvard Review of Psychiatry, 22*(2), 125–137. https://doi.org/10.1097/HRP.0000000000000032

13 We don't think the use of the word "deficit" here is the best option. Considering whether you might qualify for an ASD diagnosis can already launch a battle with stigma and your self-esteem. We encourage you to consider these "deficits" as differences instead!

Chapter 10

1 https://www.nimh.nih.gov/health/statistics/any-anxiety-disorder

2 https://www.nimh.nih.gov/health/statistics/social-anxiety-disorder

3 https://www.nimh.nih.gov/health/statistics/obsessive-compulsive-disorder-ocd

4 https://www.nimh.nih.gov/health/statistics/post-traumatic-stress-disorder-ptsd

5 Kimble, M., Neacsiu, A. D., Flack, W. F. Jr, Horner, J. (2008). Risk of unwanted sex for college women: Evidence for a red zone. *Journal of American College Health, 57*(3), 331–338, DOI: 10.3200/JACH.57.3.331-338. PMID: 18980890.

Chapter 11

1 https://www.nimh.nih.gov/health/statistics/major-depression

2 https://www.nimh.nih.gov/health/publications/seasonal-affective-disorder

3 https://www.nimh.nih.gov/health/statistics/persistent-depressive-disorder-dysthymic-disorder

4 https://www.nimh.nih.gov/health/statistics/bipolar-disorder#:~:text=Prevalence%20of%20Bipolar%20Disorder%20Among%20Adults,-Based%20on%20diagnostic&text=An%20estimated%204.4%25%20of%20U.S.,some%20time%20in%20their%20lives

5 Borgogna, N. C., Aita, S. L., Trask, C. L., & Moncrief, G. G. (2023). Psychotic disorders in college students: Demographic and care considerations. *Psychosis*, *15*(3), 229–239.

Chapter 12

1 Meaney, R., Hasking, P., & Reupert, A. (2016). Prevalence of borderline personality disorder in University Samples: Systematic Review, Meta-Analysis and Meta-Regression. *PLoS ONE*, *11*(5), e0155439. https://doi.org/10.1371/journal.pone.0155439

2 Cano, K., Sumlin, E., & Sharp, C. (2022). Screening for borderline personality pathology on college campuses. *Personal Mental Health*, *16*(3), 235–243. DOI: 10.1002/pmh.1534. Epub 2021 Dec 14. PMID: 34910370.

3 Min, J., Hein, K. E., Medlin, A. R., & Mullins-Sweatt, S. N. (2023). Prevalence rate trends of borderline personality disorder symptoms and self-injurious behaviors in college students from 2017 to 2021. *Psychiatry Research*, *329*, 115526.

4 Kiekens, G., Claes, L., Hasking, P., Mortier, P., Bootsma, E., Boyes, M., ... & Bruffaerts, R. (2023). A longitudinal investigation of non-suicidal self-injury persistence patterns, risk factors, and clinical outcomes during the college period. *Psychological medicine*, *53*(13), 6011–6026.

5 Swannell, S. V., Martin, G. E., Page, A., Hasking, P., & St John, N. J. (2014). Prevalence of nonsuicidal self-injury in nonclinical samples: Systematic review, meta-analysis and meta-regression. *Suicide and Life-Threatening Behavior*, *44*(3), 273–303. DOI: 10.1111/sltb.12070. Epub 2014 Jan 15. PMID: 24422986.

6 Schmahl, C. 2019. Neurobiology of self-harm in borderline personality disorder. ACAMH conference. London, November 8.

7 Eisenberg, D., Nicklett, E. J., Roeder, K., & Kirz, N. E. (2011). Eating disorder symptoms among college students: Prevalence, persistence, correlates, and treatment-seeking. *Journal of American College Health*, *59*(8), 700–707. 10.1080/07448481.2010.546461

8 Shisslak, C. M., Crago, M., & Estes, L. S. (1995). The spectrum of eating disturbances. *International Journal of Eating Disorders*, *18*(3), 209–219. https://doi.org/10.1002/1098-108X(199511)18:3<209::AID-EAT2260180303>3.0.CO;2-E

9 Lipson, S. K., & Sonneville, K. R. (2017). Eating disorder symptoms among undergraduate and graduate students at 12 U.S. colleges and universities. *Eating Behavior*, *24*, 81–88. 10.1016/j.eatbeh.2016.12.003

10 Arcelus, J., Mitchell, A. J., Wales, J., & Nielsen, S. (2011). Mortality rates in patients with anorexia nervosa and other eating disorders: A meta-analysis of 36 studies. *Archives in General Psychiatry*, *68*(7), 724–731. DOI: 10.1001/archgenpsychiatry.2011.74. PMID: 21727255.

Resources and Acknowledgments

Therapist Directories

- Zencare: zencare.co
- Psychology Today: psychologytoday.com
- Alma: helloalma.com
- Grow Therapy: growtherapy.com
- Therapists of Color Network: www.innopsych.com
- Therapy for Black Girls: https://therapyforblackgirls.com/
- Black Female Therapists: https://www.blackfemaletherapists.com/
- Therapy for Black Men: https://therapyforblackmen.org/
- Black Male Therapists: https://searchblackmaletherapists.com/
- Latinx Therapy: https://latinxtherapy.com/
- Asian Mental Health Collective: https://www.asianmhc.org/
- WeRNative (For Native and Indigenous Folks): https://www.wernative.org/
- Inclusive Therapists: https://www.inclusivetherapists.com/
- National Queer & Trans Therapists of Color Network: https://nqttcn.com/en/
- The Trevor Project (For Queer Teens and Young Adults): https://www.thetrevorproject.org/
- Meditationandpsychotherapy.org

Hotlines and Chat Lines

Your campus may have hotlines staffed by students or an on-call service for the mental health center after hours.

Suicide and Crisis Lifeline—call 988 or chat. A 24-hour, free, confidential suicide prevention hotline for anyone in crisis.

National Suicide Prevention Lifeline (1-800-273-TALK).

Crisis Text Line—text "HOME" to 741741. This service provides free, 24/7 crisis support via text messaging.

SAMHSA's National Helpline (USA): 1-800-662-HELP (1-800-662-4357)—A confidential, free, 24-hour information service, in English and Spanish, for people facing mental and/or substance use disorders and their families and friends.

Trans Lifeline—call 877-565-8860.

Trevor Project (LGBTQ+)—call 866-488-7386, chat online, or text "START" to 678-678.

Veterans Crisis Line (USA): 1-800-273-TALK (1-800-273-8255)—A confidential 24-hour hotline for veterans and their loved ones.

Online and On-Campus Support and Activist Groups for High School and College Students

Active Minds

Challenge Success

Healthy Minds

Jed Foundation
Kyle Cares

Parent and Family Supports

Childs Mind Foundation (for parents)
Grown and Flown
Kelly Fraidin
National Alliance on Mental Health (NAMI.org)
Understood.org

General Mental Health Support

1. **NAMI (National Alliance on Mental Illness)**
   - A grassroots mental health organization dedicated to building better lives for the millions of Americans affected by mental illness through education, support, advocacy, and awareness.
2. **Mental Health America (MHA)**
   - A community-based nonprofit dedicated to addressing the needs of those living with mental illness and promoting overall mental health through advocacy, education, research, and services.

Depression and Bipolar

1. **Depression and Bipolar Support Alliance (DBSA)**
   - Provides hope, help, support, and education to improve the lives of people who have mood disorders.
2. **American Foundation for Suicide Prevention (AFSP)**
   - Dedicated to saving lives and bringing hope to those affected by suicide, focusing on research, advocacy, and support for those impacted by suicide.
3. **International Bipolar Foundation (IBPF)**
   - Aims to improve understanding and treatment of bipolar disorder through research, education, and support.
4. **Bipolar Support Group Network (BSGN)**
   - Offers a supportive community for those affected by bipolar disorder, providing peer-led support groups and resources.
5. **Anxiety and Depression Association of America (ADAA)**
   - A leading nonprofit dedicated to the prevention, treatment, and cure of anxiety, depression, obsessive-compulsive disorder, posttraumatic stress disorder, and co-occurring disorders through education, practice, and research.

Substance Abuse

1. **Alcoholics Anonymous (AA)**
   - A fellowship of individuals who share their experiences, strengths, and hopes to solve their common problem and help others recover from alcoholism.
2. **Narcotics Anonymous (NA)**
   - A global, community-based organization providing a recovery process and support network for those affected by addiction.

3. **International Conventions of Young People in AA**
   - Organizes conventions and events for young people in AA to share their experiences and support one another in sobriety.
4. **Hazelden Betty Ford Foundation**
   - A comprehensive, leading provider of addiction treatment services, offering a wide range of recovery services and support.
5. **SMART Recovery**
   - A nonprofit organization that helps individuals gain independence from addiction through a self-empowering, science-based program.
6. **Substance Abuse and Mental Health Services Administration (SAMHSA)**
   - A federal agency that leads public health efforts to advance the behavioral health of the nation, focusing on improving the lives of individuals living with mental and substance use disorders.
7. **Celebrate Recovery**
   - A Christ-centered, 12-step recovery program for anyone struggling with hurt, pain, or addiction of any kind, offering a safe place to find community and freedom from the issues controlling their life.

Eating Disorders

1. **National Eating Disorders Association (NEDA)**
   - Supports individuals and families affected by eating disorders, and serves as a catalyst for prevention, cures, and access to quality care.
2. **Eating Disorders Anonymous (EDA)**
   - A fellowship of individuals who share their experiences to support each other in recovering from eating disorders.
3. **Academy for Eating Disorders (AED)**
   - A global professional association committed to leadership in eating disorders research, education, treatment, and prevention.
4. **The Alliance for Eating Disorders Awareness**
   - Provides programs and activities aimed at outreach, education, early intervention, and advocacy for all eating disorders.
5. **Project HEAL**
   - A nonprofit organization that provides support and resources to those seeking recovery from eating disorders, focusing on access to treatment and education.

Anxiety

1. **Anxiety and Depression Association of America (ADAA)**
   - A leading nonprofit dedicated to the prevention, treatment, and cure of anxiety, depression, obsessive-compulsive disorder, posttraumatic stress disorder, and co-occurring disorders through education, practice, and research.
2. **National Social Anxiety Center (NSAC)**
   - Aims to improve the lives of people with social anxiety disorder through public education, evidence-based treatment, and peer support.
3. **Freedom From Fear**
   - A national not-for-profit mental health advocacy organization, focusing on the needs of individuals suffering from anxiety and depressive illnesses.
4. **International OCD Foundation (IOCDF)**
   - Aims to help those affected by obsessive-compulsive disorder and related disorders through support, education, and research.

Many of the experts we interviewed have fantastic resources and books:

Lynn Lyons
Tina Bryson
Julie Lithcott-Haims
Kelly Fraidin
Jessica Lahey
Sharon Saline
Charmain Jackman
Jen Quest-Stern
Wendy Fischman and Howard Gardner

There are many schools and programs that offer significant supports, and we are listing a few we've encountered here:

Beacon College (Leesburg, Florida)—Beacon College is dedicated to students with learning differences, attention-deficit/hyperactivity disorder, autism, and neurodiversities. It offers bachelor's and associate's degrees in a variety of subjects along with support services tailored to each student's unique needs.

Mitchell College (New London, Connecticut)—Mitchell College has a focus on students with learning differences. Their Learning Resource Center offers programs and services tailored to students with specific learning needs.

Lynn University (Boca Raton, Florida)—Lynn University's Institute for Achievement and Learning offers support for students with learning differences.

Muskingum University (New Concord, Ohio)—The PLUS program at Muskingum University is designed for students with learning disabilities and other educational challenges, offering services such as tutoring, academic coaching, and learning strategy development.

Lesley University (Cambridge, MA)—The threshold program is a two-year, on-campus college experience for students with diverse learning, intellectual, and developmental disabilities.

Curry College (Milton, Massachusetts)—Curry College offers the Program for Advancement of Learning (PAL), specifically designed to support students with learning disabilities and attention-deficit/hyperactivity disorder. The program provides individualized coaching, academic support, and strategies for academic success.

Maryville University (St. Louis, Missouri)—The Life Coach Program at Maryville University supports students with learning disabilities, attention-deficit/hyperactivity disorder, and autism spectrum disorder by providing personalized coaching on academic and life skills.

Dean College (Franklin, Massachusetts)—Dean College offers The Arch Learning Community, designed for students with learning disabilities and other learning challenges. It offers a structured environment and a curriculum tailored to enhance learning strategies in addition to traditional supports.

Semester Off (Wellesley, MA)—An educational and therapeutic semester for students struggling with mental health and learning issues. Offers groups, activities, counseling, and academic supports, as well as some college credit.

Boston University—NITEO is an intensive, one-semester program supporting young adults who live with a mental health condition to develop wellness tools, academic skills, resilience, and work-readiness.

Augsburg University—The StepUP program and residence specifically for students in substance recovery with counseling and other supports.

Author Bios

Christopher Willard took six years to graduate from Wesleyan with a 2.57 GPA in 2001. He then finished his doctorate in four years. He now teaches at Harvard Medical School, where he recently won a teaching award, and has published over 20 books and spoken in 39 countries. He lives in Cambridge, Massachusetts, with his family. Chris still has dreams that he has to go back to college and take more classes to graduate.

Blaise Aguirre, MD, is Assistant Professor of Psychiatry at Harvard Medical School and an expert in child, adolescent, and adult psychotherapy, specializing in dialectical behavioral therapy (DBT). Dr. Aguirre has been a staff psychiatrist at Harvard's McLean Hospital since 2000, and he is internationally recognized for his extensive work in the treatment of mood and personality disorders in adolescents. He is the founding medical director of 3East at McLean—a continuum of care that uses DBT and related techniques to treat complex psychiatric disorders, including borderline personality disorder (BPD). He lectures regularly in Europe, Africa, and the Middle East on DBT and BPD. Dr. Aguirre is the author of multiple books, including *Borderline Personality Disorder in Adolescents and Depression* (Biographies of Disease), and coauthor of others, including *Mindfulness for Borderline Personality Disorder, Coping with BPD, DBT for Dummies, Helping Your Troubled Teen, The Unwanted Thoughts and Intense Emotions Workbook*, and *Fighting Back*.

Chelsie Green, LMSW, is a psychotherapist and holistic wellness practitioner who works in private practice. She specializes in working with young adults and the BIPOC community. Her work in private practice blends an assortment of evidence-based practices with holistic and unconventional methods. Previously, she worked as a Mental Health Educator at Wesleyan University and as a counselor in a men's correctional facility on Rikers Island. Ms. Green holds a master's degree in social work from Columbia University and a bachelor's degree from Wesleyan University, where she graduated near the bottom of her class with a 2.9 GPA and many "Withdrawals" on her transcript.

Acknowledgments

Chris: I'd like to sincerely thank my two wonderful coauthors, Blaise and Chelsie. After years of talks, we finally wrote something together. Now maybe we will actually have time to hang out! I want to also thank the dozens of experts and hundreds of students we interviewed as part of this project, and the thousands of students we've worked with over the years whose voices echo in these pages, inspiring us, and hopefully inspiring and healing you. I'd like to thank Dana Bliss for believing in the project, and Dani Segelbaum and Carol Mann for finding it a home. I'd also like to thank our family and friends, and colleagues who helped us along the way with words of wisdom and words of support. And I would not, of course, have ever completed this book or my bachelor's degree without the incredible support of family during that difficult time in my twenties, my college friends and therapists at the time who supported me, and those on the other side who showed up to walk along the path of recovery in the years since.

Blaise: First, I want to thank my coauthors. We brought very different writing styles to a shared vision, and we were able to find a way to find a single voice. Thanks to Dana Bliss, our editor at Oxford University Press who believed in our vision. To our agent, Dani Segelbaum, who was solidly in our corner throughout the process. I want to give a nod to my children,

Isabel, Anthony, Lucas, and Gabriel, who had such different experiences in college that they underscored the need for this book. But none of these acknowledgments would be relevant if it were not for the more than 15 million students who aspire to higher education each year. It won't always be easy or fun, but if you struggle with what to do, I hope that many of the ideas in this book will make your journey easier.

Chelsie: I would like to thank Chris and Blaise for being so inspiring and for all of the laughs, and Dana Bliss and Dani Segelbaum for making this book a reality. I'd like to thank all of the students, parents, and professionals who took time to share their experiences and expertise. This book wouldn't be so special without all of the voices that contributed. I would also like to thank my friends and my sister, Tyrah Green, for being supportive during the process. I have to thank Matthew Garrett, my professor and advisor in college, who helped me get through such a difficult time. I also have to thank Lisa Cohen and Sarah Mahurin, my other professors who provided me with guidance and believed in me when things were challenging. And last, I'd like to thank my mom, Kerry McDermott, who passed during the writing of this book. You never went to college like I did, but you tried your best to support me and were so proud of me, always.

We would also like to thank the following individuals:

Shannon Albarini	Lynn Lyons
Mark Bertin	Laura Markham
Michelle Bowdler	Roberto Oliverdia
Tina Bryson	Brian Ott
Nick Covino	Izi Peng
Tara Cousineau	Will Slotnick
Tim Davis	Jen Quest Stern
Jessica Grose	Nancy Rappaport
Rana DiOrio	Jason Roderick
Wendy Fischman	Jess Romeo
John Sommers Flanagan	Sharon Saline
Kelly Fraidin	Jennifer Senior
Ilan Goldberg	Jacqueline Tenaglia
Jessica Grose	Ashley Vigil Otero
Charmain Jackman	Dzung Vo
Anya Kamentiz	Jeff Waitkus
Kris Kampf	Lara Wilson
Jessica Lahey	Kendra Wilde
Broderick Leaks	Addie Wyman-Battalen
Julie Lythcott-Haims	

And perhaps most importantly, all of the anonymized students, parents, and professionals who contributed to this book!

Index